HELP! MY TEEN IS PREGNANT

HELP!
MY TEEN IS PREGNANT

A SURVIVAL GUIDE
*For Moms of
Pregnant Teens*

STEPHANIE ZEISS

NEW YORK

LONDON • NASHVILLE • MELBOURNE • VANCOUVER

HELP! MY TEEN IS PREGNANT
A SURVIVAL GUIDE *For Moms of Pregnant Teens*

© 2018 **STEPHANIE ZEISS**

Published in New York, New York, by Morgan James Publishing in partnership with Difference Press. Morgan James is a trademark of Morgan James, LLC.
www.MorganJamesPublishing.com

The Morgan James Speakers Group can bring authors to your live event. For more information or to book an event visit The Morgan James Speakers Group at www.TheMorganJamesSpeakersGroup.com.

ISBN 978-1-68350-706-2 paperback
ISBN 978-1-68350-707-9 eBook
Library of Congress Control Number: 2017912144

Cover Design by:
Rachel Lopez
www.r2cdesign.com

Interior Design by:
Bonnie Bushman
The Whole Caboodle Graphic Design

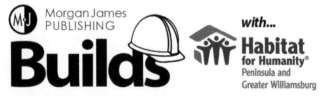

In an effort to support local communities, raise awareness and funds, Morgan James Publishing donates a percentage of all book sales for the life of each book to Habitat for Humanity Peninsula and Greater Williamsburg.

Get involved today! Visit
www.MorganJamesBuilds.com

For Brianne and Kayla,
I love you both to the moon and back!

Table of Contents

Introduction

Help! My teenage daughter is pregnant! I'm sure you never thought you would be looking for a book quite like this one. But I'm glad you picked it up. If you're hoping it would be the one to help you through this confusing and tumultuous time, answer some questions, and guide you on this journey with your daughter, then you found the right one. When my daughter told me she was pregnant at age 17, I searched and searched for the book that would help me embark on this unforeseeable journey. One that would answer some questions, give me some insight to the future, or just help me take the next step, but I couldn't find it. I ordered at least 10 books online and read them all, but they weren't what

I was looking for. Most of them were written by someone who did not personally experience raising a pregnant teen, and their stories and statistics did not resonate with me or my situation. So, after having gone through the experience myself, I decided to write it. I hope you find this book to be a comforting companion with useful information that provides some insight for you. Also included are some stories from other moms who have traveled this rough journey with their teenage daughters.

None of us really think it will happen to our daughter. We may consider it when we hear of someone else's kid getting pregnant and briefly think, "God, I hope that never happens to my kid." Or the thought might cross our mind when she comes home all googly-eyed about some boy who asked her out on a date, and she can't wait to go out with him! But, in our reality, we know she is on the right path—and that just happens to other kids, not ours, right?

The idea for this book and its title were born somewhere in the middle of my second journey. *Both* of my daughters became pregnant in high school, both at age 17, so that is not a typo above when I said, "in the middle of my second journey." I began to feel this sense of urgency to reach out to other moms who were going through this experience for the first time. I was also inspired to write it after experiencing two deaths in my family—my dad and my older sister—and then two births—my two grandbabies, all in a short period of time.

I was going through the grieving process *and* walking with my girls down this unexpected path. I felt a burning desire to get some of my experiences and ideas down on paper. I paid more attention to journaling and noting conversations I had with other moms of pregnant teens. I kept thinking that maybe someday, someone would read them and these experiences would help them too. Sometimes we go through a really difficult season of life and we need some help. I became acutely aware of how many girls get pregnant in their high school years. 17 pregnant girls, to be exact, were in my daughter's senior class! That's when I woke up to the fact that other moms were going through the same thing, and having a very difficult time getting through it while maintaining a good relationship with their daughters. I realized that my personal process, in dealing with this challenge, is sharing my experience with you. If I could help just one mom get through this with her daughter with less pain, then it was worth writing.

This book centers on helping you. This life-changing event is confusing and frustrating, and will mess with your psyche to the point of exhaustion. It would be easy to sit around feeling bad, looking for people to blame and complain to, or rehashing what you could have done differently so maybe this wouldn't have happened. Knowing this is out of your control to fix is depressing, and coping with it seems unbearable, even though you know it is the only way to the end of the journey. This book will provide some insight into the journey that lies ahead, and help you avoid the pitfalls along the way.

The chapters ahead will introduce you to some key information and skills that helped me through the difficult times with my girls. These situations tested me in every aspect: mentally, physically, emotionally, and—most of all—spiritually. I generally felt confident that I could handle anything that was thrown at me, but not this curveball. It knocked me off kilter and left me wondering: how the hell are we going to get through this? When life is going great, we tend to neglect our survival skills. I had buried mine deep down in the hollows of my psyche. I dug deep, rediscovered them with the help of my coach, and applied them during the first journey with my oldest daughter. Then I had to fine-tune them when I found myself on an unexpected journey for the second time, with my second daughter. They became "survival techniques" and a part of my permanent daily routine, and helped me become the person I needed to be throughout this process with character, wisdom, and strength.

I hope this book serves as a loving companion along the journey you are taking with your daughter. The book may serve you better if you read through it once and then go back and use it as a reference guide, mastering these skills. Study, apply, and repeat these survival skills as needed. Some days you may not need them, and other days you may be utilizing all of them. These skills are in a sense your survival "go-bag," and they will be easy to remember because they are directly linked to the word SURVIVAL.

S - Strong Mindset

U - Use Your Most Valuable Tools

R - Reconnect with Your Daughter's Needs

V - Validate Your Belief: The Baby Is a Gift!

I - Insist on Respect

V - Venture the High Road

A - Activate Your Inner Warrior

L - Love Is the Only Way

These eight survival skills help create your personal process for guiding you through this difficult time and improving your balance in these four critical areas: mental toughness (or attitude), emotional strength, physical strength, and spiritual awareness. When problems arise, we sometimes try to avoid the situation by hiding in denial, or feel bewildered because we don't know how to handle it, or handle it in a way that is more harmful than helpful. These skills will provide a pathway to handling difficult situations with ease and peace of mind. The journey ahead is not easy, so equipping your tool belt with these survival techniques is life-changing.

I hope this book helps answer your questions and replaces your fear with hope. The next couple of chapters will explain how I came to receive some of the answers to my questions through my experiences and awareness, and which areas I chose to focus on for my list of "survival skills." They will definitely help you and your daughter through this challenging time. The journey is not always difficult, but there are definitely road blocks and pitfalls along the way, and hopefully with a little insight you will be able to avoid some of the pitfalls I found myself in. We all go through difficult seasons in our life, preparing us for even greater challenges, and my wish for you is to not feel alone. You will get through this, and everyone will be OK.

Life is 10 percent what happens to you, and 90 percent how you respond to it.
— **Charles Swindoll**

Chapter 1

How I Know What I Know
About Pregnant Teens

I am a mom of two girls. Brianne is the oldest and she is 23. Kayla is still a teenager at age 19. They are both smart, beautiful girls with spunky, go-get-it-all attitudes. Brianne was a good student who marched through high school like it was no big deal. She made really good grades, seemed to like all of her teachers (except maybe her algebra teacher), and had an easy time making friends. She didn't run with a big crowd, but rather a select group of friends who all had similar goals. They liked to attend sporting events, go see movies, hang out at our house, and just do all the things happy teenagers do. She liked to tell me about things that went on at school, at her job, or with her friends or her sister. Brianne also had a steady boyfriend, but since they both had after-school jobs, they didn't seem to be all that "steady." Brianne had goals of attending nursing school after high school, and had worked hard so she could finish high school a semester early and start college sooner. She graduated in December 2011.

Two weeks before she graduated, she dropped the bomb on me. When she walked in the door, I knew something was going on with her. She said, "Hi, Mom," but she didn't really make eye contact and she kept walking past me, trying to evade a conversation.

My suspicious mom vibes kicked in. "Why don't we sit and talk for a minute," I suggested. "I've been gone a lot and I think we need to catch up on a few things. A lot has been going on lately and I need to know how you're handling it."

We were all grieving because I had just lost my dad the week before. I knew she was not handling losing her grandpa well, and I wanted to know if she needed help. She noticed that I had been crying and gave me a hug. She asked me if I was crying because of Grandpa. I said "Yes," then, with suspicious mom vibes kicking in again, asked. "Why? Is there some other reason I should be crying?"

She didn't answer right away, and I knew something big was coming. Brianne is my child who likes to tell me things. Then, after a minute, she blurted out, "I don't really want to tell you this, Mom, but I'm pregnant!"

My heart stopped, and we both burst into tears.

I didn't trust my legs to hold me up, so I just held onto her while we were both sobbing. My stomach was churning. This was the furthest thing from my mind. I told her I needed a minute and walked to the bathroom, not trusting what my stomach might do. After a few minutes of cooling my face with cold water, I came back to the kitchen, where she still sat crying. I felt like I was having an out-of-body experience. "Mom, I know you're upset…"

"Upset?" I said. "Upset is an understatement! Upset is what I am when you pull a bad grade. Upset is what I am when you stay out past curfew. This is not upset. I don't know what this is… Sick! That's what I am right now. This makes me sick! How could you let this happen? I thought you were smarter than that! What the hell, Brianne, what were you thinking? Or were you thinking? How could you let this happen? What are you going to do?"

"Mom, I didn't mean for this to happen! I'm sorry, but I really didn't think this would happen. And as for what am I going to do? I'm going to have a baby."

Denial hit me over the head. "Maybe you did the test wrong; we should probably go to the doctor to make sure," I said desperately.

She said she was already three months along and had already been to the doctor. She couldn't find the right time to tell me any sooner because my dad had been so sick, and I was away from the house visiting him. Her next doctor's appointment was the ultrasound, and she wanted me to go with her.

"So, we can't even talk about other options?" I asked.

She glared at me. "If you're talking about an abortion, you can forget it. I'm not killing my baby. If you don't want to accept this, that's fine, I'll figure this out on my own. My friends already said I could live with them if I have to."

I honestly couldn't believe that question came out of my mouth. I'm not a pro-choice person, but when my 17-year-old daughter told me she was pregnant, that suddenly became an option! I felt crazy, confused, exhausted. After about an hour of going back and forth, we started to calm down. Then, in walks her dad. We had to repeat the scene while he reacted to the news, listen to him say all the things I just said, and more.

I had to shut down the argument so we could all take a breather. This was not healthy for anyone, and a good night's sleep (yeah, right) was what everyone needed. The next day, I made an appointment with a friend who is also a family counselor. She got us in right away. That meeting was helpful and somewhat comforting. Listening to Brianne respond to the counselor's questions began to reassure me that she was mentally handling this OK. Better than me. I also learned that Brianne's biggest fear was that we would make her have an abortion, and she was already in love with her baby, so that was out of the question. Good for her, I thought. She's standing her ground and protecting her baby.

Our counselor said she was impressed with Brianne's accountability and her determination to make this work on her own if need be. She also suggested that I let my daughter walk her own path now, start releasing some of my fear that she wasn't going to be able to walk this path of great responsibility, and start trusting that she didn't just blow up her future. Brianne was capable and willing to make things work out for the best. But I had so much fear. I admitted I couldn't start "letting go" just yet.

Was I comfortable with this advice? Hell, no! This was a life-changing event. This was a life-turned-upside-down event. I couldn't just "let go"! It took a few more sessions with the family therapist to realize that what she meant was not literally letting her go … she just meant I needed to let Brianne become who she needed to be … slowly … and detach emotionally.

Now, let me introduce Kayla, my youngest daughter. She idolized her older sister most of her life. It was pretty easy for many years raising these two because whatever Brianne did, so did Kayla. They were best friends, partners in crime, and had a love/hate relationship. I thought this was awesome. When Brianne got pregnant in high school, Kayla was her sole family support until her dad and I got on board. Kayla was mad at us for reacting the way we did when Brianne told us she was pregnant. Brianne was her idol. She felt we'd screwed up, and that it was her job to protect Brianne from us.

Kayla was a good student, but didn't really care for school. It was more of a social time for her. Where Brianne liked a select group of friends, Kayla liked a group of about 300. Kayla also informed me that she was not going to college, at least not right out of high school, because she wanted to be a flight attendant. Kayla is barely 5 ft. tall, but acts like she's 10 feet tall. And bulletproof.

I was on a camping trip with my husband and his parents when Kayla sent me a text: "Mom, call me when you're not around anyone." She was supposed to be spending the weekend at a friend's house, but when I got her text I figured she had all 300 friends over for a party, and the house was on fire! So, I leashed the dog, went for a walk with my cell phone, and returned her call.

"Mom, I know you're going to want to kill me, but I have to tell you something." I was listening for the fire truck sirens in the background, but didn't hear anything. "Well, I went to the doctor, and do you remember when I switched my prescription?"

Me, warily: "Yeah?"

"Well, the new stuff didn't work, and I'm pregnant."

(Ahh … that boot kick to the gut, again.) Thank God there was a picnic bench nearby. I climbed up on it, lay down, and just stared at the stars. Again, my heart stopped and I couldn't speak. My stomach churned, but I wasn't going to throw up this time. I'd been here and done this, right? I wasn't going to react like I did with Brianne because

I had learned so much from that experience. The baby, who is now three, is the light of my life, so how can I get upset?

"Mom? Are you OK? You're not saying anything."

I said, "Umm, I just need a minute. I just need to breathe for a minute." Or maybe two or three. Then denial showed back up. "Are you sure? Your doctor said you may not have periods with the new prescription."

"Yeah, I'm sure. So is he. I went to see him before I called you. He did an ultrasound and there's definitely a baby. Are you going to yell at me now? Because I just have to say that I feel so much better now that I told you."

(Of course you feel better, but I feel like blowing up!) "No, I'm not going to yell, the campground is full. How are you doing with this? And please don't tell me it's that idiot Brad's (insert idiot's name here) baby?" Oh my God, I couldn't believe it … not again! Pregnant and 17 … the summer before her senior year!

She said she was OK, pretty freaked out at first, but she knew how much we loved Brooklyn, her sister's little girl, so her baby would be equally loved as well and that's what mattered to her. Love is the only way. Love is the only way to get through difficult life-changing events. I kept repeating this to myself as I lay on that picnic table looking at the stars. My dog had curled up next to me on the table. Well, halfway on the table, halfway on my stomach. She always knows when I need comforting. We stayed there for about 30 minutes before I decided I'd better get back before someone came looking for me. I wasn't ready to tell anyone yet, and Kayla wasn't ready for her dad to know either. How the hell was I going to get through the weekend with him keeping this secret? I needed time for myself. Time to process.

I buried myself in a good book the rest of the weekend, and told my husband I had a stomach ache and needed to lie down (at least it wasn't a total lie). I'm usually the one who likes to drag out a camping trip and push past check-out time before leaving, but not this weekend. I just wanted to be home and talking to Kayla face-to-face, so I could see her expressions and body language when she talked about her feelings about becoming a mommy. My heart was aching, and it hurt to breathe. I felt a million miles away from our comfortable, normal life. Kayla had been trying to convince me that she was alright, and that I didn't have to worry about her, but I could sense in her voice that she was scared. I had already been down this road before. I knew that there was plenty to worry about.

These two stories of my daughters and their unexpected pregnancies are still as fresh in my mind as the day they told me. There were some similarities in the journeys I took with each one of them, but also many differences. For instance: one of them was practically finished with high school (since she graduated early), the other one had a whole year to go through; one had a steady boyfriend who wanted to be in the picture, the other one did not; one of them wanted to live on her own and didn't want any help, the other one knew she needed help and a place to live. I have my own diverse experience with my own girls' teen pregnancies, as well as those of other girls and their moms who I have helped take this journey together.

We will revisit my daughters' stories and the experiences they bring to this journey in the pages ahead. We will also visit stories from other moms who have taken this unexpected journey with their daughters.

Chapter 2

Aftershock

I got to know Karen when she called me to find out more about the "moms of pregnant teens" support group I was running. Her daughter had just told her she was pregnant. She had been sitting at her desk at work when her daughter called her with the news. She said she had barely been able to walk down the hall and make it to the bathroom before she burst into tears. She was devastated. She had stayed in the bathroom for over an hour until she could get herself together enough to go back to her desk. Her daughter had just received an acceptance letter to the college of her dreams on the east coast, and they were supposed to go there for an orientation soon. She was out of her mind with grief. She was sure her daughter had blown up her future, was going to be stuck with a baby and her boyfriend, and lose sight of her goals and dreams. She felt helpless and unable to cope with the new direction her daughter's life had suddenly taken.

After the initial "shocking news," the fear is overwhelming. It seems surreal. You believed your daughter would never get herself into a situation that could potentially set her back from her goals and dreams. This isn't something she would do. Now what? What do you do from here? What is going to help? What the hell is going on? So many new questions to deal with. Everything is a jumbled mess.

Finding some information or answers to the questions that are re-playing over and over in your head will hopefully make you feel better. It's all you can focus on. Perhaps you'll find it online. Googling "why is my teenager pregnant?" "teenage behaviors," or "help for moms of pregnant teens" brings little hope that something will provide some guidance; there are plenty of articles on grim statistics and stigma-related stories, but not much in the form of support for moms who want to believe that everything can still be OK for their kids. Searching for and believing that the information you need is out there on the web is the desperate you seeking insight to this unexpected disaster. Comfort and guidance feel out of reach. There is not a plan for this; this was not expected. No one makes a plan that says, "If my daughter gets pregnant in high school, this is what we do."

Being here in this moment, thinking about what's going on and how everyone is handling it, really sucks. Your daughter is hurt because of the confrontations brought on by her unexpected news; your husband is so angry he won't even look at her right now; your other kids are upset and freaked out; and you feel like you're the one who has to make everything OK. And make *everyone* OK. You feel like it's your job to get everyone through this process without screwing things up too badly. This is what we do for our kids: figure out a solution, even if it means we never sleep again.

But what do you do first? Talk to her doctor? Tell the family? Keep it quiet until you feel better about the situation? Look for a support group? Call a therapist for your daughter and/or you? What will make you feel better about the situation? Plan a meeting with her boyfriend's parents? What are they going to think? Feel? Do?

If only you could stop this reel of questions from playing over and over in your head, but how? Until you find what you're looking for, nothing is going to make you feel better. Answers and a game plan for this new "problem" are all you want. Your daughter's pregnancy has divided the family, and everyone is hiding. Your daughter is scared and hurt and just wants to be left alone, her siblings are feeling sorry for her because they don't want her to deal with all the bullying and snide comments at school, and your husband is so grumpy, he's not even approachable. There is no peace at home. Maybe it's best to let everyone have some space.

Feeling frustrated, guilty, and full of fear for your daughter's future, you continue the Google search with things like, "Why do so many teens become pregnant?," How many teens graduate high school?," "Do teen moms go on to college?," and "College life of a teen mom." After reading a couple of articles, you realize the information may not be the best thing to soak up because many of these reports and articles err on the side of negativity; they tend to repeat the stigma that if a girl gets pregnant in high school, then most likely she will drop out, sink into poverty, do drugs, and be a bad mom, and you are not in the mood to read that. You are just looking for one article that says, "Hey, my daughter was pregnant in high school, went on to college, found a job she enjoys (or started her own business), and took her baby on her joyous journey with her." But you're not finding even a little glimpse of this vision. Now what?

Your mind drifts back to your daughter. Imagining her at school in a couple of months is painful. You wish she didn't have to go through all the bullying and judgments; you remember how badly her friend was treated last year when she was pregnant. You think about your other kids getting caught up in that drama, too. This is so upsetting. Your smart, athletic, goal-driven, college-bound girl just turned and headed in the wrong direction, or so it seems. With three little words, "Mom, I'm pregnant," everything changed. All of your expectations for her just blew up into pieces. How are you supposed to handle this? How do other moms handle this? Are we supposed to be calm and rational? Or can we just be freaked out moms for a minute? This isn't just upsetting news; this is life-changing upsetting news.

Your dream come true for your daughter has been reduced to one simple wish: that everyone will come together as a family and handle this with love and respect so the pieces get put back together and your daughter will keep moving forward. The worries keep flooding into the forefront of your thoughts that this may be more than a set-back—she will give up her goals and dreams altogether!

Going through this is much like the grieving process, and it is devastating, at first. You're grieving the loss of your young, sweet child, and praying she is going to be able to handle her new life role. How is this going to work? What does her future look like with a baby? What about college plans? All of these new questions bring feelings of insecurity. Trying to process this new information seems indigestible. The knot in your gut feels permanent, at least until you feel like your questions have been answered and some higher power has swooped down and taken all your fears away. Becoming a grandma at a young age isn't very settling. What's more unsettling is that your teenager, who is still a child herself, is becoming a mommy. Unreal. What just happened here?

The highlight reel of questions keeps running through your mind, over and over: What's in her future now? (Besides the baby, which you can't even really think about yet.) Is she still going to college? What if she doesn't even graduate high school? Oh my God, why is this happening to my daughter now? What will everyone think? These questions are mentally and physically draining to the point of exhaustion. Feeling helpless isn't something you experience often, but now you don't even know how to help your daughter get through this. How much help will she need? Where's the baby going to be when your daughter is at school or work? How much help is the daddy going to be? These repetitive questions are driving you crazy.

Also, part of the initial conversation is still bothering you: the part when she told you not to worry, she's got it all figured out. (What? Really?) She said she was OK, she wants her own family, and she will figure this out on her own if she has to. On the one hand, you admire the fact that's she's thinking about taking on all the responsibility by herself, but on the other hand you know that it is not reality. She has no clue, no reference points for this monstrous responsibility she has created, and the work/ time overload of an infant/school/job/friends scenario. You reassure yourself that what her comment really meant was: I know you're hurt, Mom, and I don't want this to be your problem.

You know she is scared too, even if she isn't acting like it. However, she's had a little more time to get used to the idea. Her friends all know, and so does her boyfriend, so she has had time to mentally process this. You haven't had any time yet; you are the last one in this group to find out. Your daughter and her friends/boyfriend have spent hours talking and fantasizing about the baby's arrival and how perfect the baby will be. Her friends have been very supportive and loving, and she may be wondering if you will be too. (After your shock wears off and you don't feel angry about the situation anymore.)

How will she feel when the baby arrives? Will she even want to be a good mom to the baby, or will it be too much for her? What if she can't stand to be a mommy and she falls into the stigmatized stereotype that society has written about teenage moms: that they are high school drop-outs, into drugs, and are irresponsible, bad moms? (No!) These crazy thoughts and questions are overwhelming and confusing. She was brought up with love and respect, and that is part of her value system now.

She needs you on her side, and wants your support. This is a long journey and the next step is dreadful. Telling everyone solidifies the reality of it. She told you how hard it was for her to come to you with it, so now telling the rest of the family won't be quite as dreadful for her, but it may be for you. Your state of denial may be protesting, "I'm not ready to tell anyone yet!" You may have a pretty good idea how certain people are going to react, and the thought of going through this is painful. A break for everyone may be a good idea. You know there will be judgments and opinions (that you would rather not hear), and people trying to make it about themselves. Taking a break from reality may be a good idea, at least for a short while until you can wrap you head around this clearly.

Christmas Break

When Brianne told us she was pregnant, a break is exactly what we needed—or maybe an escape. We decided to skip Christmas with the extended family that year. My daughter had told us she was pregnant two weeks before Christmas, so we packed up and took a trip to Colorado over the school holiday break so we could process this new information and have some fun family time before we had to start telling everyone and making this a reality. Denial is a beautiful place sometimes—especially when you're in the Rocky Mountains soaking up some clean air and breathtaking views. That really helped us take the edge off of the pain.

Here, we had an eye-opening experience. We were skiing at Keystone—yes, we were skiing knowing my daughter was pregnant, but she felt like she could handle it. She was coming down an intermediate slope and saw a small child heading toward her out of control, so she made herself fall to avoid colliding with him. As her ski turned sideways, she twisted her knee. She said she felt it pop, and found it too painful to stand. We called for the first aid sled to bring her down to the bottom of the slope where they had an urgent care/medical building. The doctor who examined her in the emergency room said she needed x-rays. We were dumbfounded! We all looked at each other like, "We have to tell him she is pregnant! No x-rays!" I didn't think the words would come out of my mouth. When I finally spit them out, he started chuckling and said no problem, plan B is a brace and crutches.

He came in later to talk to us after she was fitted for her brace and crutches, and was asking Brianne questions and joking around with her about her pregnancy, about being so young. Then he looked at me and Ron and said, "I had my first baby when I was 17; it was the best thing that ever happened to me! I'm still with my wife and we have eight kids now. My first was the blessing that started this wonderful life, and we're still a crazy bunch. Congratulations on being grandparents, I'm sure you'll love it!"

Wow! What a game-changer. There it was—the message from the higher power that said that we were going to be OK! If that guy could go on, be a doctor, and have a happy, fulfilling life after his whoops, then my daughter could go on and be a nurse and have a happy and fulfilling life, too (if that's what she wants to do). The looming vision dominated by "What's her future look like now?" just got a whole lot brighter.

We spent the rest of the vacation relaxing in the condo across from the ski resort and playing games, since Brianne wasn't very good at getting around on crutches in the snow. This was the beginning of the healing process for us, and we left Colorado in much better spirits than when we arrived.

My waning hope had been restored. And my wish for you is that somewhere within the pages of this book, your hope is restored, too.

Chapter 3

If You Could Change One Thing

The first few days are the hardest. You've chased down negative thoughts to really scary places, and the anxiety can be paralyzing. Work sucks, mind fog sets in, and you don't feel like talking to anyone, but the longer you stay in the state of denial and isolation, the worse your conditions become. All of these negative emotions that have had a tight grip on your heart muscle need to disappear, so you can start telling everyone and dealing with the reality of it with a strong mindset. So ... how do you snap out of this?

With pen and paper in hand, I'd like to introduce an exercise that is meant to provoke positive thoughts and expectations for your future. It is a goal-setting exercise, but before you start moaning and groaning about it and telling yourself you don't feel like doing this right now, hear me out. I promise it will improve your mindset. It worked for me when I participated in this exercise for the first time, and I was deeply moved by what it did for me. It was actually the catalyst that set me on a course for a new, positive life mission.

Have you ever designed a vision board for yourself, or for someone else? This is a great exercise to do when something new comes up and you need to get really clear on what your new goals are and create a game plan for how you're going to meet them. You can do this with your daughter, too, if she'll play along. This is a fun exercise and helps set things into positive forward motion. It creates ultimate goals, the big ones that cause you to really reach for them in order to make them happen. I do this with my clients, and they love it. The only difference is that I design the vision board for them after they answer a series of questions. Then I take a few days to really give it some thought and create their dream come true according to their answers to the 10 questions. The day I present their vision board to them, it's like giving them a gift! They are always very appreciative for the insight and the positive vision I created for them based on their answers to the questions. It is their dream come true.

In this case, you'll be creating one for yourself. The questions are listed below. Answer them thoroughly, with as much detail as you can, and be really honest. When creating goals, remember the sky is the limit. Don't listen to any negative self-talk or limiting beliefs you might be holding onto. When you're done, put your answers together in a story format. This exercise will focus on envisioning a healthy journey for you (and your daughter, too).

First of all, pick a category of life you would like to work on. Your choices are: Career, Relationships, Financial, Health, Spiritual, and Overall Well-being. You can choose more than one area or all six, but you'll need to answer all 10 questions for each area you pick. Then, answer these 10 questions in detail on a sheet of paper:

1. What are some of the most important/pressing goals you would like to achieve during this journey/experience?

2. What will achieving these mean to you? How will you feel? What will it look like? What will you hear? (Focus on each one of these questions.)

3. What will be different when you achieve these goals? What will you *see, hear*, and *feel*?

4. Who do you want/need to help you accomplish these goals?

5. What actions must be taken to achieve these goals?

6. What time frame do you want to set to achieve these goals? When you achieve these goals, what will be the impact on other areas of your life?

7. What skills/tools/resources do you already have to help you achieve these goals?

8. What additional tool/skills/resources will be required for you to achieve these goals?

9. Do you foresee anything that could get in the way of you achieving these goals?

10. What action steps will you take to achieve these goals?

Next, read through your answers; envision creating a story out of them. Write your story, and then read it back to yourself—out loud. You will want it sound like your own self-recorded meditation. You can even try to use a soft, soothing voice as you read it out loud to yourself. If you are having problems with this exercise, have a friend help you (or your daughter). You can create one for each other. (You may also refer to the back of the book, where I have included a couple of examples of vision statements.)

This may sound hokey, but my clients are always really impressed with the outcome. They agree that it is truly a gift when I present their vision board to them. They "see" what's ahead from a positive perspective, and can't wait to get to work on it. If you could change one thing, you'll find it here… perhaps even more!

Some people are great at goal-setting and religiously create short- and long-term goals. But for others, it may seem to be a waste of time if they are not in the habit of creating goals and then checking in on their progress. This exercise is fun and rewarding. It creates a clear picture—a beautiful story—of what your life will look like and feel like once your goals are met. I encourage you to really take some time with your answers, and create your dream come true. It is so much more effective and fun than just jotting down your top 10 goals for the year and hanging them on your refrigerator. This vision board will bring awareness to your new journey and will help you maintain a positive mindset when obstacles appear. You will feel empowered to quickly find solutions to problems when they rear their ugly heads.

One of my clients decided to make one of her goals an "emotion chart" and to check in with it daily. Her daughter was pregnant and 17, so an emotion chart was necessary and helpful. She said she felt angry all the time and didn't really know why. After we had talked for a while about some of the things going on in her life and with her daughter, she realized that what she was really feeling wasn't anger, but rather, she was just hurt. Emotions can be easily misdiagnosed if we are not in touch with them. Sometimes we are feeling guilty about something, but it may be disguised as anger. Or we decide that we are angry about something, but what we are really feeling is hurt, like my client. When these emotions seem out of control, take some time to really *feel* what you're feeling. With a little instruction and some practice, you will be able to really hone in on the correct emotion, and discover what is causing you to feel this way. Then you can diffuse it. Helping your daughter to hone in on her emotions can greatly reduce her anxiety about the pregnancy, and give her a greater sense of peace. We will go over how to do this in more detail in another chapter.

Keeping a daily journal or writing in a diary is another way to bring awareness to the emotions you are feeling. Putting thoughts, ideas, and feelings down on paper can be both illuminating and therapeutic. Include daily events and how they made you feel, too. Keeping track of events also means that you won't forget what happens along this journey! You'll be glad you did. I read over stories from four years ago and realized that events I never thought I would forget had totally slipped my mind! This is also one place you can safely express your negative feelings about your daily happenings. Getting that off your chest and on your paper is great therapy, especially at a time when you are practicing love, support, and encouragement through your daily conversations. This is where you can dump all the negative things you didn't want to air out in the open.

The next eight chapters will define eight S.U.R.V.I.V.A.L. skills. Keeping them in your "go-bag" and in the forefront of your thoughts and applying them when necessary will guide you along your journey with much more ease than if you had to take this journey without them. Our daughters are watching us and how we handle situations, especially during the difficult seasons of life. Getting through this journey with less pain, drama, and stress will take some work, but will create a healthy relationship with your daughter. She will learn these skills and how to apply them by watching you, and will have a good idea of how to form healthy relationships in the future, especially with her baby. What a great gift to give her while she is going through a very difficult and confusing time in her life!

> *A happy life consists, not in the absence ... but in the*
> *mastery of hardships.*
> — **Helen Keller**

Chapter 4

Survival Skill # 1
S - Strong Mindset

I hope that by reading through and applying some of these skills, your journey will be easier for you. The beginning is rough, but the initial shock will wear off and then you will face the question of, "Where do we go from here?" The reality of it still hurts. It's like someone came in with white paint and a brush and painted over the beautiful picture of your daughter's future—the gorgeous oil painting depicting her future plans and dreams—and erased all of them. Now, looking at the blank canvas of the future, you are under pressure to paint a new picture. You have no idea where to start. What's it going to look like? How does this baby fit into this picture? What does your daughter want now? It's hard to be creative when there is so much confusion cluttering up your mind.

In order to develop a strong mindset when stressful situations arise, I've learned to use a method called STOPA (Stop, Think, Observe, Plan, Act). It was actually developed by the United States military after years of studying survival skills and is proven to be highly effective.

Stop

You should literally sit down and stop what you're doing. When you're under stress, there are a number of physiological processes going on that inhibit your ability to think clearly, such as narrowing of your vision, auditory exclusion, a high blood pressure adrenaline dump, and much more. If you take time to sit down and stop, you can allow your body to calm back down so you can think clearly. Stopping and breathing will reboot the nervous system and calm the body down. Once you are in a calm state, you can clear out all the negativity in your mind. It's important to do this right away when you feel stressed out, and perhaps several times a day. Sitting for a few minutes a few times a day and just breathing is a great mind-decluttering exercise. (Breathing exercise instructions are in the back of the book.) Just sitting and breathing, concentrating on breathing and nothing else, will release the enormous amount of tension you've been carrying around. Your body will start to relax, and you can actually feel the stiffness in your muscles begin to fade with each deep breath. Your mind will actually feel lighter when you are done with each short session and as you make room for new thoughts and action plans.

You may also want to clear out the past few conversations with your daughter that were emotionally charged and replace them with new ones. While in the breathing session, take a deep breath and run one of these conversations through your mind—and then let it go. Breathe in again and replace the conversation with new positive dialogue. Notice the weight of sadness lifting as these old conversations disappear. When you're done with your breathing sessions, you may want to jot down a few notes about your new thoughts and clue your daughter in when the time is right.

This act of clearing your mind will help you choose to have a more positive attitude. When my daughter told me she was pregnant, I was angry. I walked around like I was dazed and confused, and like nobody had better mess with me. My mood was terrible for several days until I realized I was not acting my authentic self. As in, this wasn't like me. Walking around, snapping at people—I felt so drained being in this toxic mood. So I called my massage therapist, who couldn't get me in at the time, but who reminded me to do a breathing exercise to clear out the bad mood. You may have noticed that when you're in a bad mood, your breathing is typically very shallow. It's like your body can't function properly because it's starved of good oxygen.

So, I did what she said, and by taking a little time and breathing to clear my mind, I was able to choose to have a better attitude and keep more positive thoughts running through my mind than negative ones. Choosing to have a healthier attitude—or mindset—creates mental stability. I was able to replace my old reel of thoughts such as, "I must have failed her somehow" with "What can I do right now to help her?" Or, "I can't believe she just ruined her future," with "I can't wait to see how much joy this baby brings her." Indeed, our responses to these thoughts can transform the meaning we attach to any experience. We can't control what happens to us, but we can control how we respond to these happenings.

Staying aware of your feelings and moods takes some practice. Negative self-talk creeps in and destroys the best of moods. Sometimes if we let our mental mindset get weak, these negative thoughts creep in and we end up chasing them down to some really scary places. It leaves us feeling insecure and out-of-control. Fear is always lurking around when we are encountering something new or something big, so just acknowledge that it's there, start a breathing session, and put a new positive thought on the reel.

Think

After you've had a few minutes to stop and breathe, *think* about what you have that will assist you during this stressful time. Envisioning your journey with your daughter is one way to strengthen your mindset. Refer back to the vision board you created earlier, and remember it is meant to pave the way for your "dream come true" (a happy life for your daughter where everyone is OK). Of course, this is going to take some work, but you will then know what your heartfelt intentions are and the results you want. Did you assign a time frame to one of your goals? How about all of them? If you really focus on the big picture, you can almost see where the pitfalls and roadblocks are. Envisioning this journey and mapping out your goals will also help you release your fears of the future, let go of negative feelings that still may be lingering around, and get rid of limiting beliefs that no longer serve you. The reality of this new experience still hurts, but you have to keep moving forward. Your vision board can be your guide.

Observe

When your baby is having a baby, it's time to dive deep. Your soul may be screaming for you to leave a legacy or some contribution that will make a difference in the lives of others. Follow your internal compass on this one. Observe with great intent what it is telling you. It will help guide all of the choices you need to make along the way. It may also tell you what is missing in order to leave that legacy or contribution. Maybe your contribution is to be the best grandma to this baby. Maybe it's to just show love and support to your daughter so she is not a stressed-out mess the whole time. Does your soul long to leave behind a legacy or an imprint in the world as evidence of divine love and caring for humanity? When questions pop into your mind like, "Why is this happening to my daughter?" or "How much of this do I take on?" then spend some time with this soul-purpose exercise, and see what answers come easily to you.

This only takes a few minutes and it's pretty close to the breathing exercise from the chapter before, but with a few guided questions. As you sit quietly with your eyes closed, take in five deep breaths and slowly let them out before you start asking yourself these questions. Slowly let the answers come to you, and take a deep breath in between each question:

- Do I know what my soul's purpose is? (breathe)
- What is my contribution to this experience? (breathe)
- Can I fulfill this contribution? (breathe)
- By fulfilling my soul's purpose, will it change the lives of others around me? (breathe)
- How will it change the lives of others around me? (breathe)
- Will it change me? (breathe)
- How will it change me? (breathe)
- Will it change the world?

Whoa, that's deep! That's the purpose of this exercise, though. But it just may be that expressing love and support to this baby sends out a positive frequency to the world, and yes, you have changed it! Congratulations! You rock! How can you have a weak mindset when you know you've just changed the world and made it a better place for all humanity? You've got this!

Plan

Once you have stopped, thought, and observed, you need to make a plan with that information. Maybe the plan is to just take things one day at a time. Some may be best served by letting others assist them, while others would rather plan on self-rescue, which we will discuss in a later chapter. Once you start telling people your daughter is pregnant, some will want to assist you, and others will trigger your fight or flight mechanism. Plan on this; most people will not have the same mindset you do. They do not think the way you do, and they are not in your shoes.

If you decide to be supportive of your daughter, have her live with you throughout the pregnancy, and make sure she is comfortable and has what she needs, then don't let the "tough-lovers" try to tell you that you should kick her out because she needs to figure out her own problems. I encountered a couple of conversations with people about this. Their belief was that I wasn't really helping her, but rather enabling her, and that she'd never learn to deal with her own problems. I almost let it get to the point of argument, but then I realized they had a different mindset about it because they have not had this experience before. If they had, they would most likely be engaging in a loving, supportive conversation instead. I hope that doesn't happen to you, but if it does, just move away from these people if they don't respect the choices you make.

My choice was to help my daughter, and I didn't need anyone's permission to do that. Some people didn't agree. My daughter had a friend whose mom kicked her out when she got pregnant. Thank God there was a home for pregnant teenagers nearby where she could go live and get some help. She felt helpless and terrified. I would never want my daughter to feel that way. In fact, of those 17 pregnant girls in my daughter's class, almost half had to find somewhere else to live besides their parents' houses.

Eight or nine girls seems like a lot of homeless pregnant girls in one town, even for a mid-size one, doesn't it? Clearly, this is happening to more teens than I had ever imagined before my daughters got pregnant. We need to create a movement to protect these homeless girls. It's definitely happening to more moms and their daughters than you might think!

Act

If you do this first, you will survive: call your girlfriends first, before the rest of the family, co-workers, and colleagues. Supportive friends strengthen your mental mindset immediately, and will let you know that you are not in this alone; you are loved and supported. Maybe a trip to see them in person would be better (with a bottle of wine). With a little love, support, and encouragement, your mind will be strong enough to start spreading the news to your family, co-workers, and others who may not be supportive, and may try to judge you in a negative way. Trust your girlfriends—they will prepare you for the "non-supportive people" by lovingly joking around with you about it, all the while making sure you know they are saying things with all the love in their hearts. There is no better medicine than a good support group when things get tough with your kids. They may have some good stories of their own to share with you, too! How comforting to have those supportive people as your "rescue team" and as part of your survival "go-bag" for this journey!

Directions

There are many resources and books out there on teenage pregnancy. Many books talk about different stereotypes as to why these girls are getting pregnant. People try to make sense of what is really going on. They will write about it being a demographic problem, perhaps a poverty problem, they come from a broken home, etc. I've read most of them. When my second daughter got pregnant, I read like a fiend to try to find out why this was happening. Nothing fit. I felt like the finger was pointing in a lot of different directions, but none of them made sense to me.

The books that help the most are the ones that help you feel good about yourself, give you guidance to the next step, and help you find peace of mind and stability when you feel like you're riding the crazy train. There is a short list of my favorite reads in the back of this book.

Chapter 5

Survival Skill # 2

U - Use Your Most Valuable Tools

We all need people around who show us love and support, and during this time it is really important for your psyche that you know who your rescue team is. Unpleasant situations, events, and conversations can arise at any time, and it's good to know you have a venting outlet. If you're not sure who your support group is, you'll find out when they show up as you start telling people your teenage daughter is pregnant. It's kind of like how your teenage daughter's friends are when she tells them. Some stick around because they are your tried and true, been-through-it-all, loyal friends, and some want to leave the "unpleasant" situation, like it's contagious or something, and not want to talk to you about it. They would rather talk to others about it.

Rescue Team

Those tried and true, loyal friends become our main emotional support group, and they will help us release our fears, uncertainty about the future, and other worries that go along with raising a pregnant teen. Good friends are great at helping get rid of limiting beliefs, too. At least when you're out with your friends, you can relax in the present moment and give all those fears about the future a good night's rest. When that fear wakes up, it's like a nasty little virus, minimizing dreams and paralyzing thoughts. It can even prevent us from accomplishing goals. It sabotages our deepest desires and our heartfelt intentions. Most of us don't even realize how bad we feel until we are almost out of control. We allow our energy to drain out a little every day until we are running on empty and feeling exhausted, vulnerable, and unable to set or hold strong boundaries when we need to. When you feel yourself sinking, grab your phone. Group texting equals life support on speed dial. Your rescue team will not let you bottom out.

This team of emotionally supportive friends is very important to your survival. One of our most basic needs as human beings is to have real, authentic, and meaningful connections with other people. Studies have shown that people with healthy friendships and relationships have greater emotional well-being, live healthier lives, and even have longer life expectancies!

An emotionally supportive friendship is defined by the safe sharing of personal feelings and concerns honestly and openly, and a lack of a feeling judged by the other person. Your rescue team is made up of those who really care if you are upset, scared, worried, or happy. We need these people who are not only our good friends, but who are also good listeners and are respectful of our feelings. So choose wisely. It is rare that people have all of these qualities to lend to a friendship or relationship. I hope you are blessed with the rare ones, like I am.

Your rescue team is not only about handing you a flashlight to illuminate your darkness, or lifting you to a higher ground so you can see your way through the difficulty. Even more importantly, they are there for laughing, telling heartfelt stories, drinking wine, telling bad jokes, more laughing, not talking about something if it's bothering you, more drinking, dancing, acting silly, and staying up until 3am! If you can't do all this with someone, they are not part of your Rescue Team.

Sometimes all we really need is one person to listen to us and help us through our difficult times. Many times I listened to clients talk about their pregnant teens who didn't have family close by or hadn't established a supportive friendship group, or rescue team. I started a private

Facebook group and invited all the moms with pregnant teens to join. Some did, some didn't, but I was glad to see that the ones who didn't have an established rescue team joined and participated in the conversations. It was a comforting community for them, and helped them know that they were not alone on this unexpected journey with their daughter.

Self-Rescue

Inner strength comes not only from getting rid of toxic thoughts, but also getting rid of toxic emotions. Just like detoxifying your physical body, you must detoxify your emotional body as well. This kind of life-turned-upside-down event can bring on all kinds of toxic emotions: anger, hurt, fear, shame, sadness, as well as a combination of them. Emotional detoxing can seem like a massive undertaking, so we try to put off, like the dreaded diet. Have you ever said, "The diet starts Monday!" while you're eating massive amounts of chocolate cake? Same thing here. These emotions pile up, and they need to be released before they do permanent damage to your heart and psyche.

You can Google different methods of emotional detox, but the easiest one in my opinion is the one my coach taught me. She told me that when I was upset or angry about something, I needed to write about it in a notebook for 10 minutes. To put in as much detail as possible during that time. And then, put it away (I like to set mine on fire and throw it in the fireplace), and don't think about it again for the rest of the day. If your emotions flare up at times throughout the day, just tell yourself to forget about it for now, you'll think about it during your "worry time" and write it out. Try to limit your toxic emotional thinking to 10 minutes a day. You may need a couple of "worry times" at first until it becomes a habit. If you do this for several days in a row, you'll be amazed at how much you are breaking through these toxic emotions.

Be patient with the process; it doesn't get fixed overnight. After you have cleared your toxic emotions from your system, you can be sure that things will start to get messy again. It's just life, and once we are able to detoxify regularly, it will seem less overwhelming.

Self-rescue also means putting you first. Ha! Most moms think that the happiness of others is more important than their own. They're trying to manage all the parts of themselves that are sad, hurt, angry, and frustrated, and nothing seems to work because everyone else comes first. Why do we do this? For some women, it's because they come from a long generational female history where women's needs have been silenced by sexism or patriarchy. For others, it may be because it's a cultural belief that women are the nurturing gender, and therefore will care for their family without needing care in return. We will not go into that history, but instead will focus on what we can do from here on out. This is putting you first!

Putting yourself first means that you have respect for yourself and you stand up for what you know is right. Decide carefully about what you want to be involved in and what you don't, without feeling guilty. Moms try to always be there for their loved ones so everyone is happy, but the truth is, you can't make everyone happy, no matter how hard you try. Concentrate on those things that are important to you, and still do things for your loved ones, but find a good balance and protect your mental well-being. This will leave you with time to tend to important self-care practices, which we will go into more detail about in a later chapter.

It also means tending to your emotions. Many times I hear moms talk about how guilty they feel when they aren't doing all the things their family expects them to do. Guilt is a negative emotion, and if it is left unresolved it may lead to stress, anxiety, or depression. If you think this is what you are feeling, postpone the people-pleasing acts and tend to your emotions. Emotions are not a sign of weakness, but a sign that we are human, and they need special attention. If you detox the guilt, you will be in better mental health. We have to be in good shape to take care of ourselves and our loved ones. Ask the moms in your rescue team if they ever feel guilty about not doing things for their family, or how they find balance taking care of everyone while keeping their emotions in check. It's an important topic because now you have to help your daughter find balance, too, with the little one on the way.

Emergency Contacts

Having a coach or a therapist included in your support group will lend expert guidance when you need help breaking through these toxic emotions and working through other barriers that come up. When your whole rescue team is in force, you'll feel that "safe space." Your depression lifts, your sadness lessens, and you are back in positive thinking mode and envisioning greater possibilities for yourself and your daughter.

You may want to add high school counselors and other teachers or staff members to your extended rescue and support team. They are a great resource for information and equipped with skills that will help keep your daughter interested in high school. When things get tough at school, it's reassuring for your daughter to know that someone is there who understands what they are going through. Some high school staffers really go above and beyond to make sure these pregnant girls make it to graduation. They are more than willing to help the girls get through the day by offering to be available for them when things get really rough. I have heard many stories told by girls that some days, they would rather work on their assignments or eat lunch in the counselor's office, so they could hide out and feel comfortable at school.

The counselors will also let them know if other options are available. If your daughter is going to have the baby during the school year, the school may provide a home-schooling program that could last up to three or four months after the baby is born (depending on the doctor's recommendation). This is a unique program and allows the girls to still earn their credits and their "seat time," which is required by the district.

Here's how my daughter's program worked: Kayla had her baby in February her senior year, so the following week after the baby was born, she was assigned a teacher from her high school who would come to the house for three hours, 3 days per week, and go over Kayla's class instructions from that school day, then leave her with her homework assignments. Kayla was able to log in to the school's website and complete her homework before the deadlines. The three-hour daily appointments met the "seat-time" requirements, and the online assignments met the credit requirements.

In addition, they had certain Saturdays of the month where students could attend and make up any seat time they had missed during the week. So, if the student or the instructor had to cancel the home-school appointment because of illness or other reasons, this was an opportunity to make it up and still meet the necessary seat-time requirement for graduation. I was so thankful this program existed, because it allowed Kayla to still be able to graduate with her class. With her baby due in February, she otherwise may not have made it through, due to attendance issues with post-delivery problems: lack of sleep, baby's schedule, doctor's appointments, etc.

Think about how you will assemble your rescue and support system. Do you need to work on any of the areas mentioned in this Survival Skill #2, Use Your Most Valuable Tools: Rescue Team, Self-Rescue, or Emergency Contacts? You may want to take a few minutes and jot down some notes on what your rescue and support system will look like as you travel this journey with your daughter.

Chapter 6

Survival Skill # 3

R - Reconnect with Your Daughter's Needs

U p to this point it may have pretty easy to know what your daughter's needs are. She needed new clothes, time with her friends, time for herself in her room without mom, dad, and siblings interrupting her. She may have needed a little bit of help with her homework, a little bit of money to go out with, and some constant reminders of her curfew. Mostly, just the basic stuff. Now, things have changed, and so have her needs. She's probably still going to need all of those listed above, but with a lot more attention from you. You're her only expert in this situation, and she needs you to be available when she's ready to talk about her growing condition.

Family Communication Plan

Survival depends on having established a good communication plan. Keeping the communication lines open gets harder and harder as they become teens, and now she is really going to close up sometimes. The book by Gary Chapman called *The 5 Love Languages of Teenagers* explains how kids want to receive love and the different things you can do for them so they feel like they can be open with you. The five love languages are: words of affirmation, physical touch, quality time, acts of service, and gifts. Many families have benefitted from this book, and I know I did. I realized that my oldest daughter needed two of the five languages that are talked about in the book. She thrived on words of affirmation, and she liked little gifts. This is when she felt like she was really loved.

When our kids become teenagers we spend so much time criticizing them—you're on your phone too much, you need to study more, you're with your friends too much— that we forget to tell them all of the affirming words that we did when they were little, like "I love you to the moon and back," or "You're going to be a superstar." All of that gets overshadowed by our need to shape them into responsible teenagers, usually by nagging them. My youngest daughter felt the most love when I would just spend quality time with her. So, every day I would make sure I did something with her that made her feel special, even if it was just a half-hour trip to get ice cream, or sitting with her at the kitchen table for a snack. Being present makes a difference to them. They need to know that they have one person who will be there for them during this difficult time.

Offering to go to their doctor's appointments reassures them that you have accepted the fact that they are a teenage mom, and you support them. It is also an opportunity to talk to the doctor about any concerns you may have. Seeing the tiny body growing inside your daughter's belly is a moment flooded with emotions: excitement, love, joy, gratitude, fear, anxiety, and hopefulness. You may need to grab a tissue before entering the ultrasound room. These appointments are wide-open communication lines between you and your daughter, and the conversation lingers for days or even weeks afterwards, talking about what you saw and learned that day.

One Step at a Time

Your daughter will seem excited about the baby at times, and then others times she will feel terrified. Sometimes, they just don't think they can handle going through the birth, and then taking on the daily responsibilities of a baby, school, and friends. That's when they expect you to intervene and reassure them that they are going to be just fine. You may not believe it yourself yet, but taking it one step at a time is the only way to get her through those days of fear and worry. She may be having problems at school with bullying or losing her friends. She has put up with negative judgments from her family and friends, so it's no wonder she gets these feeling of "I'm not enough for this."

When these young girls fully accept their pregnancy, they are consumed with feelings of shame, fear, and embarrassment. I have talked with many pregnant girls who said they would try to avoid people in the hallways by hiding in bathroom stalls and stairwells. They didn't want people gawking at their growing bellies. That is why only one in three pregnant girls graduates from high school.

After reading that statistic, I was on a mission to convince my daughter she could do this. It took many long conversations in the morning, some of them tear-filled, to get her motivated to go to school. They know it's important, but they are so uncomfortable with the treatment by their peers, that they are ready to give up. They are hearing things from their peers like, "Wow, OMG, are you carrying twins?" or "She's so fat and stupid." Even "I heard she got pregnant on purpose to keep her boyfriend." This would be hard for an adult to take in on a daily basis, so just be kind to her when she's throwing a fit about going to school. A little patience, persistence, and a set of listening ears will go a long way. And when you get to exhale because you made it through the day and she's ok, tomorrow morning may be a repeat of today. This journey gets rough sometimes, so slow it down, take a deep breath, and take it one step at a time.

Flashlight

A staple in every survival "go-bag" is a flashlight. You use it to illuminate the path so you can find your way when it gets dark. In this case, you are the flashlight and you can light up the path for her. Use it when you want her to pay attention to something you're doing. She is watching how you handle yourself in certain situations, so turn it on when something important comes up and show her the way. What a great teaching moment—without preaching to her. It's good for her to be paying attention to you when you are handling difficult or adult issues on her behalf, such as when you have to address a bullying issue at school or a negative comment from a family member; what questions you ask at her doctor's appointments; and, more importantly, how you take care of yourself.

Turn it on when you want her to pick up a simple but important tip, like doing workout videos in the family room when you don't have time to make it to the gym. My daughters used to be annoyed when I'd turn on my video, and they would complain about having to deal with the loud music and instructors' voices while they were busy concentrating on their phone messages. Guess who is doing workout videos in the family room now, with the babies crawling around them because they didn't have time to pack up and go to the gym?

When I'd take a bath and stay in there for an hour reading a book with a good scented candle so I could "soak off some stress," they used to tell me I was weird. Now, guess who is sitting in tub with a good book and a candle. Yep, both of them take long baths to "soak off some stress."

Be aware they are quietly eagle eyeing you, and you could have some fun with this one. They may say that what you are doing is annoying or weird at first, but then you'll catch them doing it.

Three Points of Reconnection

After talking to many pregnant teen moms, the consensus for what they needed most from a trusted adult was acceptance, guidance, and patience. With my first daughter, Brianne, I sucked at acceptance, and made her feel bad when she told me she was pregnant, but I was good at guidance and patience. With Kayla, I was better at acceptance and guidance, but my patience would wear a little thin with her. They both tell me that they believe that if teens have these three things from their parents, educators, and friends, then they will be more successful through their pregnancies and years beyond that.

First of all, your daughter needs to feel that someone accepts her for who she is. She has to put up with so much judgment and shame that she's hoping someone will just accept her for being a teenager. Secondly, she needs guidance. Sometimes she won't act like she needs guidance or like she wants to listen to you at all, but without your persistent guidance, she just might fail. Finally, she needs patience from everyone around her. She knows she's freaking out on the inside, and so she may not be making the best decisions—or speedy ones. She needs patience when she has an attitude, and patience when she's procrastinating with homework, and patience when she wants to hang out with friends.

Regroup

When we first hear that our teenage daughter is pregnant, we think they should immediately become responsible adults and learn how to do all of the things they need to do to become a successful parent, even though it took us their entire lifetime to learn it. Time out. Regroup. Reflect on the teenage mentality. I know it's been a while, but close your eyes and think back to your own teenage years. It will help you understand that they are teenagers first and pregnant teen moms second. They are not going to get that they have to budget, find babysitters, and start college funds for their kids. Teenagers who are not pregnant can't think that far ahead, so don't expect pregnant teens to do so right away either. They will eventually come to make those decisions when their maturity level allows them to. Pressuring them about making money and budgeting for the future really freaks them out. If they are still in high school, this is enough for them at the moment. Graduating from high school when you're pregnant is a monumental accomplishment, and they need to be recognized and congratulated for it.

They will be relying on you for many things: financial support, emotional support, to be their cheerleader—the one that walks in the trenches with them—and be their babysitter when they need a break with their friends, feed their baby in the morning (sometimes) so they can sleep in, help them stay on track with school deadlines and doctor's appointments, and plan their baby shower. I hope it doesn't surprise you to find out that most teenagers do not have strong appreciation skills. They haven't had enough life experiences yet to train them in the proper use of appreciation. Appreciation, by definition, means to recognize value and significance, to be aware of the magnitude of people and things. What teenagers value the most is their freedom, and by giving all of their attention to attaining their freedom, they lose sight of the people and things around them. Appreciation for what you are doing for them and for helping them through this difficult time will come in time, but expecting it when they're still teens may leave you disappointed. Give them time to learn from their experiences how to value their surroundings and give appreciation to those that have helped them.

Be Attentive

When you're in survival mode, you must be attentive. This tactic is easy. Giving your attention to the growing baby is a great way to reconnect with your daughter's emotions. Holding her belly when the baby is kicking is really exciting. There are all kinds of tricks to get a baby to kick according to the Internet. My daughter and I tried a bunch. She would try moving around and switching positions, or she'd eat something sweet and we'd wait a few minutes. This one usually worked. Or if I'd press on the side of her belly, the baby might press back. Sometimes, I think he would just fall asleep, so she would drink a cold glass of water to wake him up, and Wham! A baby kick. It was fun to make such a production out of it. We may have worked getting that baby to kick for a half hour or so before getting a tiny result. But it was worth it, and my daughter liked all of the attention she was getting and giving to her baby.

> *When life gives you a hundred reasons to cry, show life*
> *that you have a thousand reasons to smile*
> **– Unknown**

Chapter 7
Survival Skill # 4
V - Validate Your Belief: The Baby Is a Gift

D eveloping this survival skill will fill your heart with comfort and peace. The worry you carry around about your daughter's pregnancy creeps into the first thought in the morning, and there is little you can do to keep your mind from coming back to it more than periodically throughout the day. Those questions of worry and fear keep popping up, and you try to silence them with new positive thoughts. You've told some people now and have listened to many different responses. The negative ones seem to hang around. You've heard it over and over from different people: "You know she screwed up her birth control, that's why she got pregnant. She must have forgotten to take her pill, that's just being irresponsible." Okay, maybe. She said she didn't, but that doesn't really matter now. We don't say things like, "Uncle Jim forgot to take his cholesterol medicine, that's why he had a heart attack. He could have totally prevented that." Or "Aunt Judy forgot to take her blood pressure medicine, that's why she had a stroke. If she wouldn't have been so irresponsible, she wouldn't be laid up in bed with her right side paralyzed right now."

People do say things and make up reasons for events happening so it makes sense to them. They really don't want to think that the birth control didn't work, because maybe they're on the same kind and want to keep their faith in it. So calling your daughter irresponsible is the only thing that makes sense to them. Many of them haven't taken the time to reflect on their own behavior when they were teens. They were probably doing the same things; they just didn't get caught. I know women who rarely use protection, and don't get pregnant. There are also plenty of women who would go to the ends of the earth to get pregnant and can't.

So, why your daughter got pregnant goes way beyond the fact that she made a mistake, just like any other human being, and way beyond the fact that she may be irresponsible—she is a teenager, after all—and way beyond the fact that she just wasn't thinking, or that you missed something as a mom and are blaming yourself for her pregnancy—which is crazy, by the way. She is pregnant because we all have our own unique path to walk, and this is part of hers.

Let's not forget who is really in charge of our paths that we walk in this world. Children are a gift from the Lord; they are a reward from him (Psalm 127.3). People tend to forget this important message when a teenager becomes pregnant. Society has written a strict set of rules that emphasizes that all kids will graduate from high school, and go to college. Then find spouses, have babies, and be happy. In that order. If it's not in that order, then it is viewed as failure. Do you think your daughter is a failure? Do you think you have failed her in some way? (I hope not!)

Sherry's Validation

One of my clients, who I will call Sherry, blamed herself for her daughter's pregnancy. She blamed it on herself for divorcing her husband three years previously, which meant her daughter didn't have a father figure in her daily life. She blamed herself for taking a job that required her to work more hours, even though she needed to make more money after the divorce. She felt like she was away from the house too much and not spending enough time with her 16-year-old daughter. She cried every day, believing that it was her fault that her daughter's life was now going in a direction neither one of them felt like they knew anything about because all the plans they had made for her future had seemed to go "poof into thin air." I asked her to consider how her daughter would feel knowing her mom was carrying around all of the guilt of her newly announced pregnancy.

The next time I saw Sherry, she said she'd had a conversation about her guilty feelings with her daughter, who reassured her that it was definitely not her fault. Her daughter told her she was crazy if she felt that way, and took 100% responsibility for her circumstances. Sherry agreed with her daughter that she might be a little crazy because she didn't feel much better after their conversation.

Moms can be a little crazy sometimes when it comes to our kids, and in this situation, I reassured Sherry that if she was feeling crazy, then she was definitely in the majority. She said it bothered her that she couldn't shake these guilt feelings and was almost obsessing about them. I asked her if she did any meditation or spent any time in prayer when she was feeling out of control and obsessive. She said she believed in God and she did pray, but maybe not as consistently as she thought she should and that she probably needed to go to church. I asked her if the next time she prayed, she would ask God to take this guilt off her hands. Just hand it over to him and ask him for guidance for this new path she was on with her daughter.

After a few weeks, Sherry called and thanked me for reminding her to pray. She said she also started meditating to try to calm her obsessive thoughts, and that after a couple of weeks, she was starting to feel better. She was able to release the guilty feelings that were driving her crazy. She said she also had an epiphany when she attended her cousin's funeral. Her family was not overly religious, but everyone that day was talking about God. How "this must be God's plan, to take him from his family at such a young age." Her cousin was only in his early 40s and had died suddenly of a heart attack. His wife claimed he was never sick, and had no idea he may have had heart problems. She heard more from family members: "God's the only one in control," "God must know what he's doing, but the rest of us don't," "When it's your time, it's your time." She said she kept hearing all of these comments that accepted death as God's will, the ultimate plan for her cousin.

Then she explained her epiphany: if death is accepted as God's will, then why not life? Why do people not accept a teenager with an unborn baby as God's will? If a married woman in her 20s gets pregnant, it's a "little miracle," but pregnancy was definitely not acceptable and had been viewed as something bad for her daughter! These societal rules started to not make sense to her anymore. She said she got rid of the guilt, but now she was starting to get annoyed when people would react negatively to her daughter's pregnancy (because this is an emotional roller-coaster). She said she sees her daughter's pregnancy in a different light and has accepted it wholeheartedly. She's even cherishing her new thoughts about the baby's arrival.

"Wow! What a breakthrough," I told her. Hearing the joy in her voice instead of dread was amazing. "Keep envisioning the arrival of that sweet little face. There isn't anything holier than a newborn baby!" It made me think of my two grandbabies and how they couldn't be anything but a gift.

My Validation

I'd like to share my story about why I believe my daughter's babies were gifts from God. First of all, I'd like to say that I have always believed that babies were gifts from God, but when my oldest daughter told me she was pregnant at age 17, I don't know why that belief got buried in the depths of my mind. I could not find it for the first couple of agonizing weeks of her newly announced news, and all of the family drama that came from it. I was also deeply grieving the loss of my dad, so I was not in any state of mind to hear any more "bad news." If you've experienced the grief of losing someone you love, you know that it causes a crippling pain that lasts for weeks before you even start to feel like you'll be normal again.

My dad passed a week before Brianne told us she was pregnant. I believe that my mind was not healthy enough at that point to believe in gifts, because I was almost feeling angry at my higher power. I was feeling like someone was really picking on me, and what did I do to deserve all this, anyway? Losing my dad was unbearable, but now my precious little girl is having a baby? I felt like I was drowning in grief! I kept telling myself that I could either get bitter, or I could try to get better. But really, it just came off as blah, blah, blah self-talk. I was stuck in bitter-land ... for about a month. It wasn't until I went with my daughter to her ultrasound appointment that my bitterness turned into better-ness. Seeing that tiny baby brought back my belief that babies are a gift from God, and that this was not happening to us, it was happening for us. It was an instant attitude change, and I started to look forward to the end of the pregnancy so I could hold that cute little baby.

That cute little baby's name is Brooklyn, and she filled my heart with joy the moment I held her. All of the emptiness I had been feeling from losing my dad was now replaced with abundant joy. I know she came into my life to mend my broken heart. God took my dad from us for some reason, but he also gave us this beautiful little baby to love. I am so thankful she came into our lives when she did. She was the best baby; she always seemed content, she ate and slept on a good schedule, and didn't cry much. She's now four and a half as I'm writing this book, and she is still like a little light child. Everywhere she goes, she brings joy, always smiling and having fun. People are always paying compliments about her good behavior and how happy she seems. She still fills my heart with joy when she gets to come to "Mimi's house."

Not long after Brooklyn was born, my sister passed away. She was suffering from some health issues, but no one realized she was that close to passing, since she was only 47. I felt like the grieving process was all too familiar and that it was too soon to be going through it again. My heart was broken. But although her passing caused much pain, I was beginning to understand God's will. I believed my sister was no longer suffering, and God took her because he sees the entire panoply. We do not. We only see a snapshot of our lives. Some time passed, and then Kayla told us she was pregnant. I prayed and prayed to God that he knew what he was doing with this one, because I sure didn't, and I handed over the wheel. I was able to accept her pregnancy much more easily than I did Brianne's. I didn't yell, or cry, or throw up this time, because things were making sense to me like never before. I clearly got the message that I was not in control. This was not my will. This was God's will.

I shared this awakening with my daughter, Kayla, who got a kick out of it. She thought it was cool. When I shared it with my oldest daughter Brianne, she was completely annoyed, because I didn't have that understanding when she told us she was pregnant. I tried to explain to her that some of us need to do a lot of work to reach a higher understanding of things. Having to process two unexpected deaths and two unexpected births in four years forced me into a rapid period of spiritual growth and understanding.

My two little "Mimi-babies" bring so much peace and joy to our family. Whenever I feel sad about the losses our family suffered, I am quickly reminded how blessed I really am. This validates my belief that babies are truly a gift, even when the gifts arrive early.

> *A baby is God's opinion that the world should go on*
> **– Carl Sandburg**

Chapter 8

Survival Skill # 5
I - Insist on Respect

Respect is very important in any relationship, but is easily overlooked sometimes, especially when it comes to our kids. Raising teenagers who have fluctuating emotions means that there will be outbursts at times and things will get said that are emotionally charged. Sometimes we let them slide, knowing they are just teenage hormones "out of control." Now, add pregnancy hormones on top of teenage hormones! Insisting on respect from every family member is key to surviving this journey.

Sometimes respect gets overlooked by those we are in closer relationships with because we expect them to know us and to understand us better and consequently, to also forgive us more easily because they love us. This is a time when respect should be taken seriously. There is a lot of negativity around a pregnant teen, and when she feels like she is not being treated with respect, she feels unloved. She may have more emotional outbursts because her self-esteem is low and she isn't respecting herself right now. She takes it out on you or other people in the house and disrupts the peace and harmony.

Respect means to treat someone in a considerate, genuine, and kind manner. She's most likely not getting that at school. You can show her respect by being a good listener and being considerate of her feelings when she is having a bad day, but sometimes she'll need to be reminded when her behavior lacks respect, and she may need help fully understanding the definition of respect. Sometimes kids just think that respect means to "hold the door for someone" or "be nice to elderly people." The definition of respect should reflect your home values. At the very least it should be what was already stated above, "to treat someone in a considerate, genuine and kind manner."

She also needs to know that she is valued. Some definitions of respect state that you can't really love someone if you have no respect for them. This makes sense because to be respected is to be valued as a person and have our needs taken into consideration, so how can you really love someone if they have no value to you? You can respect someone without the love component, but you cannot have love without the respect component. Teenagers tend to use respect loosely, not fully understanding the definition of respect, and it's definitely a growing problem in our society today. Helping your daughter understand the solid meaning of respect will show her how she can show respect to herself and to others as well as how to get respect from others.

What is respect? Sometimes it's easier to define respect when we are not feeling respected, such as:

- when we are not recognized
- when we are not listened to and we have something important to say
- when we are not allowed to be ourselves
- when we are being judged
- when we feel threatened by harsh words

Harsh words destroy relationships. The old saying of "Sticks and stones, may break my bones, but words can never hurt me" means that they shouldn't bother us, but words are actually very powerful! Once harsh words are spoken, they usually live on to haunt us with bitter memories.

This chapter will cover three areas of respect: respect for yourself, respect for others, and how others show respect for you. Respecting yourself can help you move forward with the confidence to make a habit of respect and share it with people around you (like your daughter). Showing other people respect is not only a critical part of maintaining important personal relationships and a great way of expressing love for them, but also will help others show respect in return. Respecting others' efforts, abilities, opinions, and authenticity will help your loved ones feel appreciated and valued.

Respect for Yourself

Respect starts with you; it comes from within. Helping your daughter learn the importance of self-respect is critical to her mental toughness right now. You may need to post a hokey sign on your refrigerator reminding her of ways she can show herself respect on a daily basis. With her growing belly, the minute she walks into school she may feel the shame and embarrassment of knowing she had sex and now every adult in the school knows she had it too. Self-esteem and self-respect disappear, and she wants to run and hide in the bathroom or her counselor's office where she feels safe. More importantly, if you're not practicing self-respect, she will not listen to you when you try to teach her how to do it.

Here is a list of things you can do to give self-respect:

- Make a list of priorities. Know what the most important things are in your life so you can make them top priority.

- Surround yourself with people who have qualities you admire, and who make you feel good about yourself.

- Keep the naysayers away from your goals and dreams. You may even want to exclude negative people from your life completely.

- Choose carefully whom you spend your time with. Do they elevate and challenge you?

- Know your boundaries. Set them clearly and stick to them.

- Diet and exercise—in order to be your best, you must feel your best. (More details in Chapter 9.)

- Book up your calendar with things you love to do, just to feel happy.

- Devote time each day to reading. The more you know, the more you can do for yourself and others.

- Take responsibility for your actions personally and professionally.

- Figure out what you stand for. You can share this knowledge with others through small acts of kindness.

- Work on reading your intuition. Trust your gut. Knowing when something doesn't feel right is important.

- Lean into what you like about yourself. Whatever your position, you can be kind and connected to those around you.

- Fight the good fight on critical issues and choose your battles wisely. Self-respect comes from knowing what battles to engage in.
- Be authentic. Live your life on your terms and live it bravely.
- Ditch any guilty feelings you may have about your daughter's pregnancy.

Just for fun, pick two items that you are not already doing and work on them this week. See if your daughter would like to participate with you. Keep notes in a journal for you and your daughter, and see how many items you can improve upon or incorporate into your lifestyles for the duration of this journey. Have some fun while developing this survival skill.

Respecting Others

Respect comes from within, so once your self-respect is fine-tuned, it will be easier to show respect to others. You will even be able to respect those that are hard to respect. Sometimes, another person's behavior is not worthy of respect, but the person is. Maybe they are just having an off-day, and can't muster the energy for anything other than being rude. Then there are those that are consistently rude and toxic, and need to be avoided in order to remain respectful to yourself. Make sure you pack an extra first aid kit in your "go-bag;" reinforcement of necessary supplies is highly recommended to avoid infection of possible wounds.

I hope this doesn't happen to you, but almost all of the people I have coached through this situation have had at least one person who really got under their skin. Why is this so common? Because you're in a vulnerable state of mind, and toxic people love to strike when they sense this. They believe they know how to fix your problems, and will insist that you listen to them for the solution.

These types of people are hard to show respect to, because they are not showing you respect when they come on strong with their opinions and try to force you to agree with them. Here are some characteristics of judgmental people. You may have an idea of who they are already, and it doesn't do you or your daughter any good if you stick around and listen to them:

1. Judgmental people are overly critical. These are not just one-time criticizers. We've all made the mistake of opening our mouths too soon and saying something we assume to be true, and then wishing we could take it back. Not the same.

2. Judgmental people criticize everyone, and over and over again.

3. Judgmental people are always jumping to negative moral conclusions. Chronic worst-case scenario thinkers.

4. They show no respect for the person they are critical of.
5. They justify what they say because they believe it to be true.
6. They are invested in the one-upmanship.
7. Being judgmental is linked with other related character flaws, such as hypocrisy, self-righteousness, insensitivity, and the enjoyment of destructive gossip.

As the saying goes, great people talk about ideas, average people talk about things, and small people talk about other people. Whatever the root cause, a judgmental person has a heart that lacks love and respect for other people. They get satisfaction out of seeing others fail because it makes them feel that they are better than the others. It is best to leave these people alone. Move far away from them, so they can't penetrate through the positive mindset you've been working on and dissolve your self-respect. You may be tempted to blurt out some obscenity to them; however this will backfire, and they will just view you as being rude and disrespectful.

Learn to identify when you are being judged (poorly) by someone. Technically, it's a way for someone to make themselves feel better, by hurting others. This is usually caused by close-mindedness and a lack of social manners. Remember this: it's them ... not you!

It's infuriating when a person who has not walked a mile in your shoes, or on your path, tries to tell you the "right" way to handle your personal situation. They will try to enlighten you with their opinion because they think they know how to do it right, even though they have no experience with what you're dealing with. If they did have experience with having a pregnant teenager, they wouldn't be judging you. They would be engaging in a loving, supportive, and encouraging conversation with you.

Same goes for toxic people: Avoid them. If you have room in your "go-bag," you may want to include a snake bite kit, just in case one strikes unexpectedly!

Toxic people are stress-inducing. Unfortunately, most of us have at least one of them in our lives (maybe even in our family). Toxic people like to violate boundaries! They are intrusive and always butting into something that has nothing to do with them, so they can try to tell you what to do. They are often overly personal, self-centered, and controlling. They like to talk non-stop, but are not good listeners and lack empathy. If they don't get their way, they will likely hold a grudge.

Hanging out with toxic people even for a short while can cause harm. You may start to lose your center because you are being slowly and quietly undermined. Their behavior is very stress-inducing and deceitful. These people will say one thing, or declare one set of values, but their actions tell a very different story. If you point this out to them, they will deny, deny, and deny any discrepancy. They will try to convince you they know why you are having these problems, why your daughter is pregnant, and the whole time their finger will most definitely be pointed at you! Do not hold space for toxic people! It's not healthy for you or your daughter. There is nothing wrong with moving into protection mode. Sometimes the best way to show respect for you and your daughter is to detach from toxic and judgmental people for the time being.

Sometimes it is very hard to show respect for some people, but for the most part showing respect means you are mindful of others' different perspectives and opinions. I only included the rant about judgmental and toxic people because I've heard this complaint over and over again, and these incidents have left deep scars on moms and their daughters.

> *You can't force someone to respect you, but you can refuse to be disrespected.*
> – **Unknown**

Ideal Ways to Show Respect to Others

- Be a great listener; this sounds easy, but to truly listen is a skill worth developing.
- Be encouraging—show them you care.
- Remember feelings matter. Be mindful of other people's feelings, it may mean everything to them.
- Be positive. Positivity gains respect.
- Genuinely express appreciation, and be specific and positive.

- Express your love. Respect is one of the most meaningful expressions of love.

Ideal List for Your Daughter

- Ask to use someone else's stuff.
- Consider the way you speak to people: tone, words, body language.
- Accept others' differences as OK and legit.
- Live within the boundaries that have been set.
- Avoid gossiping and insulting others.
- Listen and accept feedback.
- Pick up after yourself.

And add anything else you can think of that might support your family values. Also, encourage her to set goals and make plans for achieving them. Each goal she sets and attains will give her strength to challenge herself to achieve more. The more goals she attains, the deeper the respect grows. Working on all of these will help her develop a well-rounded sense of respect for herself.

Getting Others to Respect You

Respect will come naturally to you if you are respecting others, and showing respect for yourself as well. The first two sections on respect are the most important for this time in your life while you're on this journey with your daughter. But here are a few other things you can do to gain respect from others that you may want to try:

- Gaining respect by practicing generosity.
- Being a role model and walking the talk. People respect those who inspire them to be their best.
- Being good at what you do. Everyone loves and respects competent people who are the best at what they do.
- Honoring what you say. This builds trust and integrity, and allows you to play on the field with your highest self.

Having respect in your house is the primary concern. Make sure everyone is being respectful so the relationships with the ones you love aren't damaged by harsh words and acts of unkindness. Respect outside of the house is also important, especially for you and your daughter's emotional well-being. Not always do our best efforts bring forth the results we want, but we lay a foundation for what is acceptable and what is not. Stick to the boundaries you set around respect; it will help them have success with their current and future relationships.

Chapter 9

Survival Skill # 6
V - Venture the High Road

The high road is love. The low road is fear. You know what it's like to be on the high road. You feel high and nothing fazes you. You feel full of patience, understanding, and connected to the world. You also know how the low road feels: full of stress, exhaustion, resentment, and the sense of always having to be right.

You've respectfully listened to everyone's opinions and judgments and decided to take the high road. This means you feel like you're doing the right thing, even if it's not the popular choice or if it's not easy. Giving yourself permission to wholeheartedly accept your daughter's pregnancy and helping her through the process feels like a rite of passage. You may even want to come up with your own ritual that celebrates the beginning of your new role. Or buy yourself a little gift (for the "go-bag") that symbolizes the new beginning of your unexpected journey. You've heard the negative opinions of others, and it doesn't feel right to punish your child for making a mistake. She's punishing herself for it enough and is looking to you for help and guidance.

What are the other options, anyway? Kick her out and tell her she's on her own? Make her marry the guy who's the father of the baby? Some people believe that is the best way to handle the situation, because it will "make her grow up and learn from her mistakes." It doesn't mean anyone is wrong for believing that; everybody has the freedom of choice, whether we agree with them or not. But just imagine for a minute that you decided to kick her out. You kicked your daughter out, and now where is she living? What is she doing, with her schoolwork, job, and social life? Is she eating enough food? Are they healthy choices? Is she scared? Will she call you if she is? How is she surviving? Does she have survivor skills?

The few girls I had the privilege of talking with who had to find other places to live after they got kicked out for being pregnant told me they were so afraid at first, but that they also understood why their parents did that. They'd let their parents down by having sex when they knew their parents wouldn't approve, and they were resigned to having to figure it out and pay for their mistakes on their own. They were amazingly brave girls. They were really thankful for the help they'd received from other people: a church group, a friend's mom, a relative. They'd found a way to get some support during a really difficult time, and appreciated those who'd helped them. They all agreed that finishing school was the hardest part, and wished their moms had been there for them. One of the girls graduated from high school, and the other two dropped out their last semester and completed their GED online. Good for them! They toughed it out through a really difficult time and still completed their high school requirements or equivalent.

What kind of relationship do you still want with your daughter? Making the decision to help her may have been an easy one for you, or maybe not? Most of the moms I have talked with were not ready to let their girls go and fend for themselves. Others needed a little time and a little soul-searching before making the right decision. Sometimes, it was the husband who wanted to kick the girls out and make the baby-daddy be responsible for the situation "he got her in." You feel the weight of the work-load ahead, but maybe there is no other option that's right for you. This decision needs careful consideration, because I have seen marriages dissolve because of this.

Sometimes it takes the dads of the pregnant teens more time to get on the high road. This is their little girl and they are struggling to handle the new life/role changes their daughter is going through because of "some boy." They can't take the high road because they feel like their survival skill is to stay at the camp and defend their family from "wild creatures." They may grumble and act unapproachable for what seems like a really long time, but they will eventually come around. You don't have to wait for that either. Your daughter needs you on board, first and foremost, so venture the high road alone for a while if you have to.

Anne's Road

I met with Anne, whose daughter was pregnant. Anne was at a crossroads. She wanted her daughter, Shelley, to stay and live with them so Anne could feel like she had some control over her daughter finishing high school, and could make sure she was keeping herself healthy throughout her pregnancy. Her husband, on the other hand, did not. He did not want the financial responsibility of another child, nor did he want to have to devote his time to a baby, and he didn't want his wife to be saddled down with a newborn (wild creature). I asked her how her relationship was with her daughter, and she told me they were very close and this was an easy decision for her to make. She couldn't imagine not helping her daughter, because she loved her and wanted to make sure she finished high school. She also wanted to make sure she had things she needed, like good nutrition and clothes for her growing body. But her husband didn't want this. He was really disgusted by his daughter's behavior and was not willing to be open-minded about helping her.

I asked her how the relationship had been between Shelley and her dad, and she said that Shelley had been on a rebellious kick for about the last six months, and he had threatened to kick her out a few times before if she didn't straighten up and improve her grades. She said he had even told Shelley a few times that the way she was acting, she was going to end up pregnant or something stupid like that, and once she'd actually gotten pregnant, he felt that she needed to be punished for her behavior. He also felt that he and Anne didn't deserve to be punished for Shelley's behavior. So he was unwilling to help her.

I asked Anne to talk to her husband and find out what kind of relationship he would like to have with his daughter. She said she would talk to him and see if maybe he had cooled down a bit and could think about being more supportive. A couple of weeks later, she came back and we talked some more about her situation. She said it had actually gotten worse because his family was backing him up and he was in no mood to put up with Anne telling him that he needed to be supportive. When she asked him what kind of relationship he wanted to have with his daughter, he said he wished things could have been different, but now Shelley had made her bed and so she just had to lie in it.

Anne felt sick about her husband's perspective and couldn't understand how he could just toss out the child they loved so much—especially at a time when Shelley needed support from her parents the most. She said it was really causing a lot of arguing and tension around the house and something had to give. Anne realized that it was in her power to change the situation. She talked about getting her own place for her and Shelley, she made plenty of money for that, but then she ultimately realized that she just needed to focus on her own wants and beliefs. She decided that when her husband started an argument, she would take the high road and say to him, "I love my daughter, she is not going anywhere," (and walk away). If it meant he would be the one to pack up and leave (which he wouldn't), then so be it.

Anne told me that after about a month of saying her mantra whenever he was ready to pick a fight, it started to work. Shelley was no longer acting like a rebellious teenager, and had turned her energy and her focus onto her schoolwork. She still avoided her dad as much as she could, but he had also stopped picking at her and asking her when she was leaving. At the time I am writing this book, Anne is planning Shelley's baby shower. Shelley still lives at home and is doing well in school. Dad is coming around, maybe not wholeheartedly yet, but he is learning to accept Shelley's pregnancy and the fact that she needs love and acceptance from both of them.

Giving yourself permission to wholeheartedly accept your daughter's pregnancy may not be as easy as you think. It may take some soul-searching through prayer or meditation to help you decide just how much help you can give her. She will need help financially and emotionally, and it can be draining sometimes. So prepare yourself for the extra help you will have to provide once you make this decision. Reward yourself for making this decision. It will take more of your energy, time, and money, so make sure you are taking care of yourself and putting your needs and your health first. This is not an easy journey for either of you, but if you are in full strength when problems arise, and they will, you will be able to give her the extra help she needs without feeling drained. Venturing the high road and wholeheartedly accepting your daughter's pregnancy is like seeking higher ground and finding shelter on this unexpected journey ahead.

Chapter 10

Survival Skill # 7

A - Activate Your Inner Warrior

M aking the commitment to walk side by side with your daughter on this wondrous, mysterious journey is empowering. You may also now be aware of how much energy it will require from you, and that it is time to focus on fine-tuning Ms. #1. Your mind fog is clearing up, and thoughts are feeling a bit more positive. You've made the decision to help her with her needs, and now is a great time to make a plan to take care of your needs too. It's time to fine tune some of those "self-rescue" practices that have been on the to-do list for a while. There are hundreds of ways that you can show yourself love and respect so you can feel better than you ever have before. Why not? You're getting ready to have a baby in your house, and you're going to be a ... grandma! (Cringe, right?) I hope at least one of your friends calls you Glamma because you know you're much too young and hot to be a grandma.

If you've been out of the self-rescue practice for a while, here are some great tips to get you back into the swing and make yourself feel like million bucks.

Bootcamp
First of all, take a look at your schedule and see how you can squeeze in 90 minutes of Me Time every day (or at least five days a week). This is the get-the-body-moving-and- stronger portion of the self-rescue plan. Try to break up this 90-minute plan into two intervals throughout the day. You could:

- Take the dog for a 30-minute walk in the morning, and attend a one-hour yoga class in the evening.
- Move along with a 30-minute stretching video in the morning and have a one-hour weight-lifting session with a personal trainer in the evening.
- Put in 45 minutes on the treadmill in the morning, and play 45 minutes of racquetball or another favorite sport later in the day.

The point is: all you need to do is fill in two intervals of time each day (at least five days a week) on your calendar with some type of exercise that is going to get your body moving and make you feel good about yourself. Figure out what your bare minimum would be, and don't let anything (like excuses) take you under the minimum. For example, one of the moms I coached figured she needed to improve her muscle strength. At our age (haha) we should be concerned with keeping our muscles toned and strong. Weight lifting also improves bone density, and will help you burn more calories on a daily basis, so she said her bare minimum was three one-hour sessions of weight lifting per week. Then she added in time for exercise classes on the days she wasn't weight lifting. She added a swimming class and two yoga classes per week. Then she was going to fill in the rest of the time with short, 20- to 30-minute walks whenever she could, at least three days a week. She thought that it would be easy to meet her bare minimum with that schedule. So with her three hours of weight lifting and three hours of exercise classes plus one to two hours of walking per week, she got in seven to eight hours of exercise. At first, she didn't think she could devote that much time to her workouts. 90 minutes a day sounded like a lot to her. But when she broke it down in terms of the week, it didn't seem like that much. Eight hours a week fine-tuning her body became do-able. Some health experts claim that you only really need 20 minutes a day for exercise. That's great for some people, but this journey you're embarking on requires strength and fine-tuning, and 20 minutes a day isn't going to get you warrior-worthy.

Nutrition

Next, take a look at fine-tuning your eating habits. Including lots of fruits and vegetables along with lean meats will keep your body in calorie-burning mode. Nobody wants to cut their favorites foods out of their diet, but if those foods are carb- or sugar-loaded, they will not make you feel at your best, and you may want to keep those in smaller portions and limit to once per week. I'm not suggesting a strict diet, but if you're working out, then your body needs nutritious foods so it will perform better for you and help prevent you from exercise injury and muscle fatigue.

I have included a list of resources in the back of the book if you would like any additional information on nutrition. Not only have I listed books on nutrition, but other books that can take you through complete body workouts. For example, the book *Goddess to the Core* by Sierra Bender talks about a four-body fitness program (physical, mental, emotional, and spiritual bodies). There are quizzes for each body, and you can quickly gauge where your fitness level is in each one and prioritize your workouts from there. Here are few more warrior-worthy tips that only take minutes to complete and you can squeeze them in at any time:

- Put on your favorite song and dance for a few minutes.
- Inhale an upbeat smell; peppermint reduces food cravings & boosts mood.

- Pick out something from your closet that feels good on your skin.
- Have a good laugh. Call a girlfriend or family member you have fun with.
- Take a power nap. 10 to 20 minutes can reduce sleep debt, and energize you.

You can Google body care tips and get many, many more ideas. Create a body care plan with as many little tidbits as you can to keep you feeling good throughout the day.

Relax (You've Got This!)
You may find that keeping your mind clear and focused along this journey will be something of a chore. Fears creep in, problems your daughter may be having will weigh heavily on your mind, and dealing with negativity can be mentally exhausting. If you haven't tried meditation yet, it may be something to consider. There are plenty of resources online that demonstrate how to get started with this mind-calming exercise. I have also included a few resources in the back of the book.

When you meditate, you focus on your breathing or on a visualization while sitting calmly. For some people, it is an exercise that helps reduce stress and promote relaxation. It can also help put a stop to racing thoughts that are causing you to be distracted. For others, it is more of a spiritual practice to promote awareness of the present moment. This may take some getting used to, but it is a quick mind-calming exercise that anyone can do almost anywhere. Some people devote only 10 minutes a day to this exercise and claim to have fantastic results. There are also recorded meditations that are available to listen to when you have a few minutes. Grab a meditation CD for your car if you have a long commute to and from work.

Reading is an excellent way to get your mind off of your worries. There are so many good books out there that will just sweep you away from all of your problems for a while, and take you on an adventure. Relaxing in a hot bath with a good book is like a mini-vacation. Books also travel well; they can be a good companion on lunch break or when you are traveling on business. Books provide information and make you smarter. They tell us stories about people we don't know and take us to places we've never been. Reading stimulates your mind and awakens your imagination, keeping your mind fresh. Studies also show that reading more books improves focus and concentration, makes you smarter, reduces stress, and improves memory. So, there you go Glamma, a great memory-builder!

Rescue Team Revisited!

Also, consider finding a good coach or therapist. There will be times that you may need some new insight, or a fresh perspective in order to solve a problem. The key is to keep your focus on the solutions, not the problems. Sometimes we get stuck in the problem and need a little guidance to get back on track. Having a good coach or therapist means you will have the support you need to sharpen your problem-solving skillset, and to set your inner warrior into action.

A few more warrior tips that will only take minutes to complete are:

- Be selfish. Do one thing today just because it makes you happy.
- Unplug for an hour. Switch everything to off and get away from the alerts.
- Scratch a lurker off your to-do list.
- Write in your gratitude journal. Try for five things you are grateful for each day.
- Goof off for a bit. Tend to your sense of humor.

Plan some warrior activities and put them on your calendar. These are also important for your overall health.

- Schedule a massage (at least 90 minutes).
- Schedule a dentist appointment or eye appointment if you need one.
- Schedule a mani/pedi.
- Plan a weekend getaway with your friends.
- Plan a night out dancing.

By regularly scheduling these small pleasures into your busy schedule, nothing will seem quite as difficult as it did before. Indulging in these self-rescue practices will help you feel more connected to yourself and your world. Also, these practices can help us avoid health problems due to stress. By improving our mental and physical health, we will also be improving our self-esteem and overall well-being. These practices can help us create a lifestyle that keep us healthy, happy, and more in tune with our mind and bodies. Remember your daughter is watching you. If she sees how well you take care of yourself, she will eventually want to do that for herself as well. Showing her that it is important to love yourself and treat yourself well is a great gift to give to her, especially at a time when she needs some extra love and attention.

I have come to believe that caring for myself is not self-indulgent.

Caring for myself is an act of survival
*– **Audre Lorde***

Chapter 11

Survival Skill # 8
L - Love Is the Only Way

I saved the best survival skill for last. If you can keep your heart full of love along this journey (even when you're really fuming), you will be aware of all of the little blessings that come with it. If you can see your daughter through the eyes of love, you will see her in a different light that no one else can see. If you know that love is the only way, then you know you will get through this unexpected journey and everyone is going to be OK. Your love will lift her to higher ground so she can see her way through the difficulties, help her feel confident to fend off the wild creatures that cross her path, and will feel like her protective gear when she's feeling alone.

By honing these survival skills, especially this one, you may feel like you've created your own protective gear and can slip into it on a moment's notice. If you've been applying these skills so far, you will be able to handle some of the unexpected potholes that go along with this journey. Learn to expect the unexpected so you can be adaptable when situations arise. Be prepared for these biggies! These are the ones that create a crisis and you will need to send up a flare and alert your rescue team. (Don't forget STOPA!)

Quitting School

This one always comes up. Even the girls who are honor roll students and absolutely loved school before they got pregnant will contemplate quitting school. At least that's been my experience. Every one of them said the same thing: that at first they thought it would be easier to just quit school. This is an emotionally charged statement brought on by fear, and they all go through it in the beginning. When they drop the bomb on you, be prepared for your emotionally charged reaction.

They have seen other girls who were pregnant before them go through all the teasing and bullying, and they don't want to be next. Dropping out and getting a GED online is really enticing to them. Some girls have moms that don't think that's such a bad idea, and that their daughter's mental state during this already difficult time is more important than their high school diploma; but if you are who I think you are, the statement, "Mom, I'm just going to drop out" will press your panic button.

When you hear these words but before you say anything, take a really deep breath in … or two or three … and then calmly ask her if she's really thought this through, or is this the easy way out. She will probably go into an explanation about how school sucks and all of her teachers treat her badly now that they know she's pregnant, and all the kids are teasing her, and she doesn't want to do it any more. You may want to agree with her that it must totally suck, but before any rash decisions are made, a clearer picture of her day should be established.

Here are a couple of questions that you may want to ask her:

1. What are the names of the teachers that are treating you badly? You want names! Ask her to write the names on a piece of paper.
2. Who are the *all* of the kids who are teasing her? Again, you want names on paper.
3. Are there any kids who are supportive and still friendly to you? (Even if it's just one.)

When she's finished (and it may take a while, because she really wants her truth to be heard so she can quit school) and looks at the (tiny) list, she will see that it's not that many people. Try asking her specific questions about each name on the paper.

How well do you know this person? Why does it bother you that this person made your "everybody hates me" list?

What does this teacher do specifically to make you think they are treating you badly? How is your grade in this class? Are you on time for class? Are you paying attention (or falling asleep) in class?

She may not want to answer all of these questions but will appreciate you sticking with her and thinking this through. What usually happens is the list of "all these people" boils down to about two or three, and then it's easier for her to understand who she really needs to avoid, and who she can count on for support throughout the day. Taking it one step at a time is a concept that needs constant reminding not only for you, but for her too. She may need daily pep talks; and she's arguing every point you make; she's tired, she doesn't feel good, everybody hates her, but you somehow convince her to go. It's really hard to see our daughters leave the house for school with tears streaming down their cute little cheeks. One step at a time.

Absenteeism

Taking it one step at a time may go well for a while, but then the bottom drops out. She left for school on time, but a couple of hours later the school calls and says she isn't there and they need an excuse for her absence. "Ummm…

well? Let me call her and see what's going on. I know she left on time. I'll call you back." You also know she is a bundle of nerves and is probably letting all of her fears get the best of her right now. Hopefully she not sitting in her car alone somewhere bawling her eyes out. Maybe she just went back home and back to bed after she knew you left for work. You can bet that every day while driving to school she is contemplating driving right past the school's parking lot and on to better things.

This will most likely happen, and it is a concern. Absentee policies are pretty strict these days, and it would be good to know how many days she can miss a class before she loses credit for it. With the upcoming doctor's appointments and other pregnancy-related legitimate reasons for her missing school, skipping is a red flag. It can make or break her school year. This is very upsetting because you know that her state of mind is not wrapped around the fact that if she sets herself back, and doesn't graduate on time or with her class, it's only going to make finishing school worse. You know she'll feel worse and more like a failure if this happens. She isn't going to want to go the following year, and face even more judgment and teasing, so her probability of dropping out increases.

Look, some days are really rough. But if she knows you are there for her and encouraging her to do her best, it's all you can do. She just has to believe that you're going to get through this, and when she does graduate, it will mean even more to her that she stuck it out, and you were always there for her, even on her worst days, to make sure her ass was in that seat when it needed to be.

Falling Grades

If this happens, it's probably due to one of three reasons, or maybe all three. First of all, it may be due to absenteeism. She may have missed a study session for a big exam because she had to go to the doctor's office for an appointment, or maybe she was legitimately sick that day. Pregnant girls get sick a lot, probably due to the stress they're going through, so you let her stay home due to her illness, of course not knowing she was missing a study session. A big, fat "F" on an exam can really hurt a quarter grade.

Another factor could be that she has foggy focus. She is so concerned with being pregnant and what everyone thinks, her focus in school gets really blurry. She forgets to turn in assignments, or to bring the right book home to study for an exam, or doesn't remember homework instructions and does an assignment completely wrong. A few missed assignments in one class can really pull a grade down. Usually kids can make it up, but not if she isn't paying attention to deadlines. Sometimes they need help with deadlines. I know teachers who will email the parents if a student has missed an important assignment or has a few missing and the quarter is almost up. It's a blessing if your daughter's teachers are willing to do this.

The third reason may be her attitude towards school. If she is putting up with bullying on a daily basis, she may feel like school is a waste of her time because she is starting to believe they are right, and that she should just drop out. This one is the hardest to detect and the most difficult to overcome. If her grades start falling, then become a detective and figure out what's going on. Sometimes it's as easy as asking the right questions, and other times it may require additional help from a professional with her self-esteem. If her grades keep falling, so does her self-esteem.

Some Friends Disappear

This is a given. Friends will quit hanging out with her because it may be an uncomfortable situation for them to be associated with her and her growing belly. She will accept some of them leaving, but when it's a friend who's been around for a long time, she will be heartbroken and so will you, because you know how badly she is hurting inside from being dumped. She may be feeling really insecure, knowing her so-called supportive friends are dwindling and, in her mind, the bullies are becoming more numerous. Put on your coat of armor and tell her how important she is, and that these friends are really missing out on having a good person in their life. Some of them may be gone forever, but some of them will reappear after the baby is born.

She's Sick … a Lot

We all know that pregnancy is difficult, and it should be. Growing another human being inside of your body is not supposed to be easy. She may have morning sickness, afternoon sickness, and night sickness. She will most likely not want to do any chores, since she went to school and her after-school job that day. She doesn't feel like doing homework … ever. She may not even want to socialize with her friends very much anymore. That coat of armor comes in handy when you're trying to encourage her to get some things done and she ends up in tears because she is really just hormonal and her moods swing continuously. Remember, she is a teenager first, with all of her teenager hormones and then the pregnancy hormones pile on!

Difficulty with Family Members

Expect the unexpected in your own home 24/7. This is a life-changing event and the whole family is dealing with it. Sometimes they're not dealing with it very well. Her siblings may feel hurt, shamed, or embarrassed for her at first. They may have emotional outbursts at home and get into fights with her. Sometimes siblings can be really messed up about it at first, until they've had time to get used to the idea. One of the pregnant girls I talked to said her older sister got so angry that she moved out after they had a fight. Her sister said she couldn't stand how stupid she was for getting pregnant.

Sometimes the harshest judgments come from those you love the most, and it's very painful when this happens. Refereeing these emotional events is difficult because both parties feel like their feelings are not being validated or that you're playing favorites. You see the pain everyone is going through, and it feels out of control. Everything has changed. Everyone has to deal with it, no matter if their behavior is acceptable or not. Things will calm down. This is one of those pitfalls along the journey, and they want you in the pit with them.

This survival skill #8—Love Is the Only Way will protect your health, mentally, emotionally, and physically. Knowing that these problems may arise will give you time to prepare for a solution instead of a reaction that may cause you more harm than good. Over-reactions are stress-inducing, and may leave a feeling of anxiety for days or weeks. If you are not on your game for days or weeks, nobody else will be either.

If mama ain't happy, ain't nobody happy.
– Unknown

Chapter 12

Insight to Additional Obstacles

Applying these eight S.U.R.V.I.V.A.L skills throughout your journey with your daughter will empower you to help her and plan for the "unexpected." Of course, most of us can't see into the future, but having gained a little knowledge by reading what others have gone through before you will lend a little insight to the obstacles that may come up, and will assist in planning strategic solutions. Being able to foresee what events lie ahead is a big advantage in our behavior and our responses to different problems, enabling us to protect ourselves from health triggers such as panic attacks and emotional outbursts that may leave us feeling vulnerable and drained. Having organized discussions about a few additional obstacles that could arise may help everyone feel more in control and more confident that you will get through this and be OK.

Your Daughter's Boyfriend/Co-parenting

Up to this point, it's been all about you and your daughter and how you will get through this journey and feel good about her future. Now it's time to consider another important factor in this situation: her boyfriend. How does he fit into the picture? Is he interested in being a part of the baby's life, or is he claiming this is not his baby? How are you going to handle communication with him from here on out? What are your daughter's expectations about their relationship?

Teen fathers are treated differently partly because a teen pregnancy is viewed as the woman's issue. She is the one carrying the child, and so her sexual behavior, intelligence, and her maturity are questioned by her peers and other adults around her. The father escapes the judgment, being treated more as the teenagers they are and not necessarily the fathers they will become, so this may delay his acceptance of fatherhood. He may be in denial and thinking about how he can avoid being around your daughter and her family at first.

However, if they are seriously together, then they may be planning to live together once the baby is born. Perhaps the thought of starting their own family isn't all that scary for them, but it terrifies the hell out of you. Where will they live? How will they take care of themselves and the baby? You know it's a huge stretch; it's probably not even possible for them to get their own place yet. Both of them having only part-time jobs and not making any real money are the first concerns that fuel your disbelief. Where is the baby going to go when they are at work? Daycare is expensive. She may want you to be the caregiver when she is at work. How would that fit into your schedule? Oh, and heads up! Your daughter may also want her boyfriend to move in with you!

What would you do if she asked you if he could move in to your house so they could have a better shot at being together as a family than they would if they had to do it on their own? Or maybe his parent(s) want to help with the baby and he wants her to move in with him. How would you feel if she wanted to live with him and have his parents help with the baby? What would be the ideal solution for you? What or how much are you willing or able to give in order to help her with the baby?

She May Not Have a Healthy Pregnancy

As a mom of a pregnant teen, this is going to be a worry. According to a few doctors I have talked to about teenage pregnancy, most girls in their teens have very healthy bodies and very rarely develop a problem with their pregnancies. This contradicts most of the articles on the web about teenage pregnancy. These articles focus on problems such as low birth weight and complications of the mother's pregnancy and birth due to lack of prenatal care. However, the doctors who have delivered babies to teenage girls have a different story. They claim that since their bodies have not yet been polluted with alcohol, smoking, drugs, or bad food (or at least very little) young women give birth to the healthiest babies. They also say that if the young moms did have a history of smoking, and alcohol and drug abuse, they were at a higher risk for premature labor and child birth. However, they very rarely see a problem with the development of the fetus, so I wouldn't spend too much time worrying about a serious issue.

However, checking in on her prenatal care will help you feel more confident that she will be OK and so will her baby. Simple things such as getting enough sleep, taking her daily vitamins, eating plenty of fruits and vegetables, and drinking enough water throughout the day will improve her overall health both mentally and physically. If she's fueling her body well, she will be able to meet the demands of pregnancy and may have some energy for light exercise, which will help her feel good about her body and boost her mood.

Out of 100+ girls that I have talked to, I only know of two that had complications with their pregnancy in late term. Statistics say one in a hundred. In both cases, the girls were neglecting their prenatal care at first, and not taking very good care of themselves, either.

Julie's Story

Julie didn't find out she was pregnant until she was late into her fifth month of pregnancy. She was a heavy smoker and had a history of drug abuse. She did not have a supportive family background, and had dropped out of high school and completed her GED her junior year. She was living in an apartment with a friend and working full-time. She said she was on the birth control pill and that is why she didn't realize she was pregnant until she started to get "fat" well into her fifth month. She was totally shocked when she found out and scared. She knew her lifestyle may have damaged her baby. She quit doing drugs, but could not give up the cigarettes. Her baby was born early at 30 weeks, weighing in at only 2.5 lbs., and had some breathing difficulties. Her baby had to be fed through tubes and remained in the hospital for three months until her breathing difficulties cleared up. At the present time, the baby is five months old, still a tiny little thing, but thriving, growing, and happy.

Crystal's Story

Crystal's background was similar to Julie's. She was raised in an abusive household and spent most of her junior year bouncing around, living with friends or in her car. She dropped out of school her senior year to work full-time and shared a small apartment with her boyfriend. She also had a history of smoking and drug abuse, although she said it was recreational drug abuse, and not addiction. She was excited when she found out she was pregnant because now she would have someone to love wholeheartedly, and she swore she would never treat her baby the way her parents had treated her. She quit all of her bad habits upon finding out she was pregnant, and decided to take care of herself. In her seventh month of pregnancy, she developed a condition called complete placenta Previa, and the birth was considered high risk. The high risk concern was for Crystal, not her baby, because the placenta could tear and present the possibility of uncontrollable bleeding. Her C-section went well, but as they predicted, she had uncontrollable bleeding for six hours after birth. Her baby was also born with breathing issues, which were corrected within a couple of days. Her hospital stay was extended as well, but only for a few days.

In both cases, the girls had insurance through Medicaid and were happy it was available to them because they would have been saddled with astronomical hospital bills and it would have taken them years to pay them off.

Medical Bills

Even if you have good insurance and your daughter is covered under your policy through her pregnancy, there are always going to be deductibles and copays that the insurance does not cover. Knowledge is king. Discussing this situation with your insurance company and asking detailed questions about coverage will help you understand what to expect and/or notice when a bill may not have been paid that was supposed to be covered. Once the baby is born, the baby will need his own insurance. Your doctor's office or your insurance company may be able to guide you in the right direction to finding a policy for the baby, or your local child services office will help inform you of the possibilities of Medicaid and WIC, depending on your circumstances. The baby will need the insurance at the time of birth, so you or your daughter do not get billed for medical costs that may exceed your means.

Stigma

The stigma of being pregnant in high school lasts well beyond the high school years. It means your daughter may have to be relentless about fighting society's judgments long after the baby is born. Teen moms are typically associated with being high school drop-outs, living in poverty, doing drugs, being single moms, and being bad moms. All of these stereotypes can cause a lot of harm if she lets herself get bogged down with them and allows them to determine what kind of mom she wants to be. It's something the parents of teen moms will have to defend against as well. Mostly the stigma is completely annoying, because it comes from those who have never experienced the walk we have with our girls, and sometimes it comes from those you least expect it to.

Robin's Story

Robin is a young grandma and traveled the teenage pregnancy journey with her daughter two years ago. Last year, during Lent, she went to a fish fry with her husband and her grandbaby, Kylee. She loves spending time with Kylee and says she tries to "steal" her as much as possible. She can't believe how well things have turned out since her frightful days when her daughter was pregnant. They went through the food line and were having a problem finding a couple of empty chairs, when the priest invited them to sit with him and some of his friends who were fellow parishioners.

During the conversation, the priest referred to Kylee as Robin's daughter. Of course, she corrected him and said she was grandma. He said she looked way too young to be a grandma. She jokingly said that since her daughter was a young mom, she graciously made Robin a young grandma. And she told stories about how much fun and joy Kylee brought to their family. He proceeded into some sort of homily about "God's children," and they talked long after their meal was finished. She had explained to him that they were supposed to meet their friends there who belonged to the church, but something had come up at the last minute and they had to cancel. She also told him that she didn't really claim a denomination as far as religion goes, but she had grown up in a Lutheran family, and had not attended church on a regular basis in several years. She didn't want to explain to him that her spiritual journey had led her down a God-seeking path in other ways besides going to church.

Upon leaving, he invited them to join their church and told Robin that if she brought God back into her life, things would start looking up for her. She said she didn't understand what he meant by that. She didn't think she let on about any negative things going on in her life. He said he meant that she would be on a path with God and wouldn't have to worry about things happening to her like her children having illegitimate children, and she should encourage her daughter to do the same thing, so she would learn the importance of celibacy before marriage.

Robin told me she thanked God her jaw had dropped to the floor so she couldn't respond right away. Her husband gently put his arm around her and guided her away from the table before she could unleash her fury on the priest. She concluded that she would never join that church or go back to support a fish fry in the future. The struggle with stigma is real.

The obstacles listed in this chapter were only mentioned to give a little insight into some of the problems others have experienced along their journey. Some who have traveled this journey with their daughters didn't experience any of the problems mentioned. However, if you feel you are having a difficult time and need more help, I hope you seek out a good relationship coach or therapist in your area. I also provided additional information for you, which you can access through my website listed on the Thank You page at the end of this book. I wish you and your daughter a safe and happy journey!

Chapter 13

Conclusion

S ome studies show that teenage births have been declining for the past decade, but the United States still holds the highest rate. This seemed odd to me when I read it, but then I started wondering why that might be. Could it be that we teach our daughters to be independent, strong women? Encourage them to make decisions, stand up for what they believe in, even if no one agrees with them? Before I took the journey with my oldest daughter, I had a misguided belief that girls who got pregnant in their teenage years must have a problem with their self-esteem, or come from an unsupportive family and feel like they were cast out only to find love on their own.

That old belief couldn't be farther from the truth with my two kids. When my second daughter got pregnant before her senior year, I went on a mission to figure out why this may be happening to my kids and some of their friends. I read numerous books and most of them had the stereotypes and the old belief system that I once had. Reading all of those books didn't fulfill my mission, so I decided to open my eyes to a bigger world and saw just how many girls become pregnant in their high school years.

The girls I've had the pleasure of speaking with during their pregnancies seemed down-to-earth, had good heads on their shoulders, and were ambitious, goal-oriented, smart, and fearless, with a strong desire to be independent. None of them felt like they were pressured into sex in general, or unprotected sex in particular. In fact, most of them believed they were protecting themselves in some fashion. They just never dreamed it could happen to them. For them, making the decision to have sex was their *own* decision, one they felt mature enough to make and to handle the consequences of.

So, moms, they were not thinking about all of those lectures you gave them about having sex, or unprotected sex—in fact they were not thinking about you at all at that moment in time. They don't want you to feel any guilt; you didn't miss anything as a parent. Sometimes they grow up way too fast, and we are not ready for it. They really aren't ready either, but they do want to feel supported, not shamed;

accepted, not rejected; respected, not disreputable; and loved, not neglected.

If you really want to empower your daughter to be a strong, independent woman, then walk the walk through this journey with her. Show her how strong women handle difficult situations with support, acceptance, respect, and love. She needs someone to validate her feelings, and you are the first in line. You have the strength and knowledge to lead her through this. You may want to go back through this book and make sure you have all eight of these survival skills properly placed in your tool belt. The road gets pretty rough at times, but if you're using and applying these skills, they will make the journey much easier for you. Remember your S.U.R.V.I.V.A.L skills!

S - Strong Mindset

U - Use: Your Most Valuable Tools

R - Reconnect with Your Daughter's Needs

V - Validate Your Belief: The Baby is A Gift

I - Insist on Respect

V - Venture the High Road

A - Activate Your Inner Warrior

L - Love Is the Only Way

Practicing or applying all of these skills will allow you to laugh at society's stigma, and you will never let it wear you down. It may not feel good right now, but there is goodness on the horizon. Both times I have taken this journey, I have found joy along with the pain, and the bumps in the road always presented a hidden lesson or blessing. The end result is always a blessing. I hope your journey with your daughter is filled with excitement along with the bumps, too, and soon you will believe that you will get through this and everyone will be OK.

Breathing Exercises
Techniques for Relaxation and Managing Stress

Tips

Ideally, sit with your back straight.

Place the tip of your tongue against the ridge of tissue just behind your upper front teeth, and keep it there through the entire exercise. Exhale through your mouth around your tongue. Try pursing your lips slightly if this seems awkward.

STEPS

Exhale completely through your mouth, making a whoosh sound.

Close your mouth and inhale quietly through your nose to a mental count of 4.

Hold your breath for a count of 7.

Exhale completely through your mouth, making a whoosh sound to a count of 8. This is one breath. Now inhale again and repeat the cycle three more times for a total of four breaths.

The absolute time you spend on each phase is not important, but the ratio of 4:7:8 is important. If you have trouble holding your breath, speed the exercise up but keep to the ratio of 4:7:8 for the three phases. With practice, you can slow it all down and get used to inhaling and exhaling more and more deeply.

This exercise is a natural tranquilizer for the nervous system. Unlike tranquilizing drugs, which are often effective when you first take them but then lose their power over time, this exercise is subtle when you first try it, but gains power with repetition and practice. Use this new skill whenever anything upsetting happens, but before you react. Use it whenever you are aware of internal tension. Use it to help you fall asleep.

How often? Do it at least twice a day. You cannot do it too frequently. Do not do more than four breaths at one time for the first month of practice. Later, if you wish, you can extend it to eight breaths. If you feel a little lightheaded when you first breathe this way, do not be concerned. It will pass.

Mindful Breathing Exercises
3 Yogic Breathing Techniques

UJJAYI

*****Contraindications: avoid this technique if you are experiencing irritation of the throat or sinuses.*****

- Sit up tall and relax your abdomen.
- Allow your belly to move with each breath.
- As you breathe, gently contract the back of your throat so that you are making a soft, continuous hissing sound like the sound you hear in a seashell. Do this on both the inhalation and exhalation, and keep your mouth closed the whole time.

- Continue the deep breathing and explore how loudly you can make the sound, but do not strain. Focus all of your attention on the sound of your breath.

- Continue this breath for several minutes, or until you start to feel calm.

- When finished, sit in stillness and quietly feel the effects.

NADI-SODHANA

- Sit up tall and relax your abdomen.

- Take a few deep breaths to calm the mind.

- Close your right nostril with your thumb, and slowly inhale through your left nostril.

- As soon as you finish inhaling, close your left nostril with your ring finger and exhale through your right nostril.

- As soon as you have exhaled through your right nostril, inhale through your right nostril. As soon as you finish inhaling through your right nostril, close it again with your thumb and exhale with your left nostril. Continue this pattern (exhale, inhale, switch).

- After several minutes of breathing in this way, begin to slow down your inhalations and exhalations. Do this very gradually. As the meditative quality of your practice deepens, you will be able to breathe even more slowly. Let the slow pace be a reflection of your mind slowing down.

- When you are ready to end your practice, release your hand to your lap and exhale through both nostrils. If you are doing complete rounds, you will finish by exhaling through the left nostril.

- When finished, sit quietly for a few minutes and feel the effects.

KAPALABHATI (advanced technique)

*****Contraindications for this breathing technique include pregnancy, recent surgery, injury or inflammation in the abdominal or thoracic region, and uncontrolled high blood pressure. If you have any of these conditions, skip this advanced breathing technique, and enjoy the benefits from the techniques mentioned above.*****

- Sit up tall and relax your abdomen.
- Take a few deep breaths to calm the mind.
- Inhale deeply.
- Strongly contract your abdomen, exhaling sharply through the nose.
- Allow your abdomen to relax from the contraction so that a passive inhalation happens.
- Repeat exhalations and inhalations at a steady pace. If you find that you become short of breath, feel light-headed, or lose your rhythm, slow down

and make sure you are taking in enough air on the inhalation. It takes some practice to coordinate the breathing with the movement of the abdomen. Rest when you feel tired.

- Finish with an inhalation, and then exhale and hold out as long as is comfortable.

Vision Statement
Example 1

Emily, after finishing your morning meditation and exercise, you sit down at your desk and take a deep, cleansing breath in… and get prepared for your busy day. You begin by answering the queries you received from your clients and accepting the registration requests for the online course you designed and launched back in March. The course is aimed at helping parents deal with their teenage children addicted to drugs and alcohol, a cause that is close to your heart. It has become your mission in life and your goal to reach out and help the families you compassionately identify with. You take another deep breath, and as you are about to respond to an email, you pause, and briefly reflect on how you started this wonderful, fulfilling career. As you gaze out the window that faces your beautiful garden, your thoughts take you back down memory lane.

What used to be a life filled with fear and mental illness is now in the past. You know now that all of the struggles were meant to teach you how to serve others with this rapidly growing problem, and the process of serving others has healed you. It hasn't been easy, but your passion to help others has finally come to fruition. You couldn't be happier with the "new you."

You have strengthened your self-confidence with the coaching and counseling you've received, but more importantly, you got where you are today through perseverance and hard work. Your self-care practices, meditation, and determination empowered you to become the woman you've always dreamed of: one that doesn't give up on her goals. You've built the lifestyle you've always wanted by becoming a life coach. You've also built it quickly by learning the "ins and outs" of social media … you've launched your company's webpage, started a blog, and created Facebook ads. You are no longer challenged by technology, but instead are in control of it.

Your first speaking engagement really got your business rolling. It was the first time you had to speak in front of a large crowd. You still can't believe you lived through that experience! You were terrified, but in the end, it was a victorious day. You overcame your fear of speaking, and with confidence and passion, you successfully delivered your inspiring speech to a large, cheering audience. It was exhilarating to hear all the cheering and clapping coming from the audience—especially from the first row, where your husband and kids were seated. It was the sound of acceptance, an acknowledgement of your success, and the feeling of fulfillment. You have become an empowered woman who helps empower others to overcome mental illness and has built her own successful business. This is your dream come true.

You take a deep breath and raise your eyes to your laptop screen, intending to start the day's work, when you notice an email message in your inbox. After some hesitation, you click on the message and read it, and then read it again and again. All you can see is, "We will grant you…," and all you can hear is your heartbeat getting stronger by the minute. Another victorious day! The donors have agreed to give enough money to start your own facility!

You walk calmly away from your desk, get yourself a cup of coffee from the kitchen, and walk out to your garden, where you sit on your rocking chair feeling relaxed, collected, confident, and successful. Life couldn't be better. You are touched and blessed once again with this last piece of your initial goal achieved. Your own facility!

Nothing can stop you now, because you are no longer a dreamer, but an achiever. You expanded your coaching business to enjoy greater financial benefits; you created an overwhelming demand for your newly designed online courses to help parents with their troubled teens—one of several ways you will touch and change the lives of many—and are in the process of expanding your reach even farther. You enjoy the wonderful feeling of achievement and confidence of a well-established wellness coach. Your upcoming speaking engagements no longer terrify you. You know your message is so important to those who need your help, and your efforts have raised public awareness of the issue beyond your wildest dreams.

You take another deep breath in and with a smile on your face, you head back to your desk thinking, "And my next goal is…."

Vision Statement
Example 2

Tammi, as you close your eyes and take a deep breath in, you'll feel your body start to relax from your head to your toes. Allow yourself to visit that safe place, that all-knowing place that resides inside you. Take another deep breath and ask your soul to be present with you. As you feel yourself relax, you begin to acknowledge yourself for the things you have accomplished. Acknowledge yourself for the skills you have developed, the businesses you have built, and how you've triumphed through a very difficult time in your life. Acknowledge yourself for achieving your soul's highest desires and goals! You are so fulfilled by your accomplishments! Tell yourself thank you for showing up and becoming the person you dreamed of.

Breathe in slowly, and notice how nice it is to just be in the present moment, taking care of you. You have all the love and guidance you need within yourself, and you trust it. These changes you have made recently have made your soul soar, and everything is crystal clear now. There is no more confusion.

You open your eyes and look around, and feel that you are overflowing with gratitude: your wonderful son just kissed you on his way out of the door for school, your beautiful home envelops you with a sense of peace and comfort, and the people around you love and adore you. You feel God's light and warmth on your face while sitting in front of the picturesque window in your living room.

You close your eyes again and breathe in slowly, returning to that safe, secure place. You begin reflecting on your achievements once again, knowing that you are following your soul's vision and that everything has come together for you. You've worked hard and put together a tool belt of skills that has allowed you to leave a legacy and imprint on this world. Through your coaching and counseling, you have built your businesses to levels beyond your wildest dreams. Your clinics throughout British Columbia are thriving and expanding! The hospital for PMF that you and your team created is healing more patients than you ever dreamed of. And your book, along with your coaching business, is helping more people with colitis disease than any doctor has ever done. You have nurtured your soul, and you have been rewarded.

You take another deep breath in, and you can't help but notice how much energy you have right now. Your new exercise routine has been so much fun that you don't ever think about missing a single day of it. Getting out and enjoying nature and all its beauty is so revitalizing, and connects you to your source of power. Your head is screaming, "Get your shoes on, let's go!" But your heart says, "Finish your meditation … there's more to be thankful for … then go!"

You sink further into your safe place, breathe in deeply, and realize that so much abundance has come into your life and has allowed you to become an Angel Investor. It has also allowed you to embark on the trip of a lifetime … with your son! You express your gratitude for having the time and freedom to travel to different countries with your message of PMF, and you get to take your son with you! You envision what it's like to show him what true service is all about. What a gift!

Your feelings of well-being are at a new height. You feel completely balanced. You have finished your transition from difficult times and have learned from the lessons that presented themselves: lessons of forgiveness, seeing your truth, and calling out your own BS. You are comfortable with your new perspective on life and acknowledge full acceptance of what is and what is meant to be.

You take one last deep, cleansing breath in and let your mind float back to the people in your life that have helped you the most through this period of change. You thank each and every one of them for their love and support. Your son, for being such and awesome eight-year-old; your mom for editing your book and helping you get it published and out to the public. Your business partner, who helped you launch new clinics. And the new man in your life, who is not only loving, kind, and supportive, but encourages you to be your authentic self. He mirrors your vision of being true to yourself, and supports your vision of leaving a legacy. A legacy built not only for your son, but for the world, to benefit from your knowledge and diligence and provide a better method of healing.

You are calm. You are relaxed. You feel alive. Open your eyes. Wiggle your fingers and toes. Notice how great you feel. Now, get your shoes on, and go!

Further Reading

The 5 Love Languages of Teenagers, by Gary Chapman
Dear Mom (Diary of a Teenage Girl series), by Melody Carlson
Dial Down the Drama, by Colleen O'Grady
Things I Want My Daughter to Know, by Alexandria Stoddard
5 Conversations You Must Have with Your Daughter, by Vicki Courtney
It Was Always Meant to Happen that Way, by Brooke Castillo
Goddess to the Core, by Sierra Bender
Girl on a Swing, by Nancy Kennedy

The Meditation Bible, by Madonna Gaulding
The Universe Has Your Back, by Gabrielle Bernstein

Good Reads for Health and Nutrition:
The 17 Day Diet, by Dr. Mike Moreno
Eat Right for Your Type, by Dr. Peter J. D'Adamo
The Blood Pressure Cure, by Robert E. Kowalski

Acknowledgments

I have dedicated this book to my two girls, Brianne and Kayla, for creating the journeys that led to the birth of this book, and for opening my eyes to a bigger world and recognizing the need for this message to be let out of my body! I love you both with all of my heart.

To my grandbabies, Brooklyn and Holden, who made me believe in God's purpose. Your cuteness melts my heart every day.

I am grateful to my mom and dad (my dad who now resides in heaven) for always encouraging me to be my authentic self. I appreciate your patience and persistence through the years I was not listening, but I finally got the message.

A big hug and thank you to my hardworking, handsome husband for sticking out this wild rollercoaster ride with me for the last 24 years!

To my girlfriends and sister: Cynthia, Mindy, Kim, Cindy, Linda, Shari, Becky, Tracy, Shannon, and Jacque. I couldn't have made it through the journey without all the laughs, trips, and wine! Thank you for all the support and encouragement. I love you all!

Thank you, Adrienne, for inspiring me to find a stronger connection to God and the universe. Through your spiritual healing I was able to love myself for who I am and become a stronger, fiercer woman.

To Angela Lauria, for creating such an awesome writing process and encouraging this author-in-transformation with your powerful training and honest feedback!

To the Morgan James Publishing team: Special thanks to David Hancock, CEO & Founder for believing in me and my message. To my Author Relations Manager, Margo Toulouse, thanks for making the process seamless and easy. Many more thanks to everyone else, but especially Jim Howard, Bethany Marshall, and Nickcole Watkins.

And to all of the moms who contributed their stories and gave me permission to interview them for this book, thank you for the group therapy!

About the Author

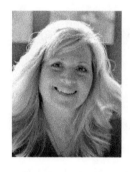 Stephanie Zeiss received her BSBA from the University of Missouri-St. Louis. She has worked in the field of health and wellness for many years as a certified fitness trainer and yoga instructor. She is also a Certified Life Coach who specializes in helping women with their teenage daughters. She lives in Missouri with her family and likes to spend quality time with her two grandchildren.

www.momofpregnantteens.com

zeissmart@yahoo.com

Thank You

Hi! Thanks for reading *Help! My Teen's Pregnant: A Survival Guide for Moms of Pregnant Teens*. I hope the book serves you well and provides you with peace of mind throughout the journey with your daughter.

Please feel free to visit my website and download a free checklist to help you stay the course: www. momsofpregnantteens.com

You may also register to receive the free audio series that goes along with this course and sign up for a sample class from the Moms of Pregnant Teens program!

If you were struggling with your vision statement from Chapter 3, please email me at zeissmart@yahoo.com. I'd be happy to schedule an appointment with you and get that done!

Sending much love to you!

Stephanie Zeiss

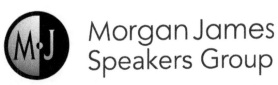

Morgan James
Speakers Group

www.TheMorganJamesSpeakersGroup.com

We connect Morgan James published
authors with live and online events
and audiences who will benefit
from their expertise.

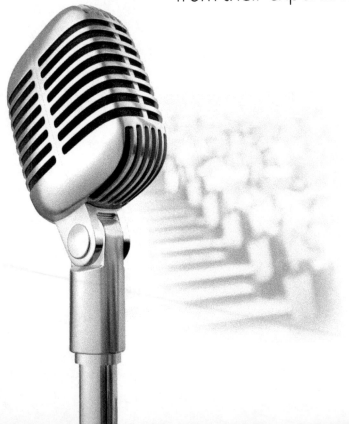

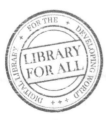

Morgan James makes all of our titles available
through the Library for All Charity Organization.

www.LibraryForAll.org

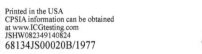